201 Skin Cases
Diagnosis & Treatment

201 Skin Cases
Diagnosis & Treatment

Fourth Edition

Sanjay Ghosh MD
Former Professor and Head
Department of Dermatology and Venereology
MGM Medical College and LSK Hospital
Kishanganj, Bihar, India
Former Medical Director (Honorary)
Institute of Allergic and Immunologic Skin Diseases (IAISD)
Kolkata, West Bengal, India

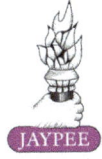

JAYPEE BROTHERS MEDICAL PUBLISHERS
The Health Sciences Publisher
New Delhi | London

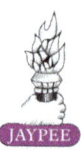 **Jaypee Brothers Medical Publishers (P) Ltd**

Headquarters
EMCA House
23/23-B, Ansari Road, Daryaganj
New Delhi 110 002, India
Landline: +91-11-23272143, +91-11-23272703
+91-11-23282021, +91-11-23245672
E-mail: jaypee@jaypeebrothers.com

Corporate Office
Jaypee Brothers Medical Publishers (P) Ltd.
4838/24, Ansari Road, Daryaganj
New Delhi 110 002, India
Phone: +91-11-43574357
Fax: +91-11-43574314
E-mail: jaypee@jaypeebrothers.com

Overseas Office
JP Medical Ltd.
83, Victoria Street, London
SW1H 0HW (UK)
Phone: +44-20 3170 8910
E-mail: info@jpmedpub.com

EU GPSR Authorised Representative
Logos Europe, 9 rue Nicolas Poussin
17000, La Rochelle, France
Phone: +33 (0) 6 67 93 73 78
E-mail: Contact@logoseurope.eu

Website: www.jaypeebrothers.com
Website: www.jaypeedigital.com

© 2024, Jaypee Brothers Medical Publishers

The views and opinions expressed in this book are solely those of the original contributor(s)/author(s) and do not necessarily represent those of editor(s) or publisher of the book.

All rights reserved. No part of this publication may be reproduced, stored or transmitted in any form or by any means, electronic, mechanical, photocopying, recording or otherwise, without the prior permission in writing of the publishers.

All brand names and product names used in this book are trade names, service marks, trademarks or registered trademarks of their respective owners. The publisher is not associated with any product or vendor mentioned in this book.

Medical knowledge and practice change constantly. This book is designed to provide accurate, authoritative information about the subject matter in question. However, readers are advised to check the most current information available on procedures included and check information from the manufacturer of each product to be administered, to verify the recommended dose, formula, method and duration of administration, adverse effects and contraindications. It is the responsibility of the practitioner to take all appropriate safety precautions. Neither the publisher nor the author(s)/editor(s) assume any liability for any injury and/or damage to persons or property arising from or related to use of material in this book.

This book is sold on the understanding that the publisher is not engaged in providing professional medical services. If such advice or services are required, the services of a competent medical professional should be sought.

Every effort has been made where necessary to contact holders of copyright to obtain permission to reproduce copyright material. If any have been inadvertently overlooked, the publisher will be pleased to make the necessary arrangements at the first opportunity.

Inquiries for bulk sales may be solicited at: jaypee@jaypeebrothers.com

201 Skin Cases: Diagnosis & Treatment / Sanjay Ghosh

First Edition: 2005

Fourth Edition: **2024**

ISBN: 978-93-5696-921-6

Dedicated to

My wife Shrabani

Regarding this Book

- The primary aim of this book is to judge the clinical acumen. The book, however, does not ignore the importance of investigations by laboratory and other methods, which may be necessary in many clinical situations to confirm diagnosis, assess degree of severity, and find associated features.
- The target readers of this book are MBBS undergraduate students or practicing physicians who have not done any specialization in dermatology. Hence, common skin diseases have mostly been described, but some uncommon and major dermatological cases signifying serious prognosis or systemic involvement demanding immediate referral have been included as well.
- Treatment guidelines represent only a sketchy plan to treat the individual case described which may require elaboration in certain cases and may not be applicable to all similar cases.
- Only standard conventional treatment mentioned in the authentic textbooks or journals have been mentioned omitting therapies which are not much evidence-based.
- Standard dose of the drugs has been mentioned which will, of course, depend on body weight, other concurrent medications, liver and renal status, known drug allergy, etc.
- Pre-therapy and post-therapy monitoring of drugs by laboratory tests should be done whenever required.
- This book does not insist that all the cases should be managed by nondermatologists. The book has attempted to provide a basic visual knowledge for diagnosis of certain skin disorders along with basic management strategy for the primary-care physicians. Referral to a dermatologist seems to be desirable whenever a situation arises.

Preface to the Fourth Edition

A lot of demand from the readers, students, and practitioners has inspired me to again bring out the new edition of this book. I have not only updated the previous information and data in light of newer knowledge and advancement of medical sciences but also included another 50 new cases for the students. Hopefully, this will create genuine interest among the readers and they will be enriched by the newly added contents. I thank the whole team of Jaypee Brothers Medical Publishers, my dear publisher, who have been motivating me for the last few years to rewrite the book and supporting me out-and-out for the present edition. Because of my hectic practice and academic schedule, I could not complete the job earlier. Last but not the least, my labor and effort would get fulfilled only if the book turns out to be helpful for those who are the chief target of this book.

Sanjay Ghosh

Preface to the First Edition

Dermatological training is often inadequately executed in MBBS undergraduate and post-MBBS internship days which leads to the qualifying remarks either "too difficult" or "very simple" regarding the subject "Dermatology" by some qualified doctors in their practice. Some feel interested but are very much apprehensive about diagnosing and managing even an easy case confidently. Some consider the subject by oversimplification and diagnose each ring-shaped case as a ringworm or tinea. They never find any depth in dermatology! Many others are totally indifferent about the subject. Of course, there are large numbers of physicians who, even without any specialization in the subject, have acquired the unique skill to deal with skin cases adequately and confidently.

Whatever may be the attitude of the physician toward the subject, each and every doctor, whether practicing or nonpracticing, has to face and even treat dermatological cases in certain situation. Hence, doctors should have some basic concept about the subject of dermatology so that they do not take the cases casually. They may not manage the case but they should know when to refer the patient to prevent fatality.

Another myth regarding the skin cases is that skin cases neither kill nor are cured. Yes, skin cases can cause life-threatening situations such as Stevens–Johnson syndrome (SJS), toxic epidermal necrolysis (TEN), erythroderma, drug hypersensitivity syndrome, pemphigus vulgaris, bullous pemphigoid, and malignant melanoma. Scabies, by secondary infection, may lead to acute glomerulonephritis, a fatal condition if not treated promptly. Manifestations of some of the serious systemic ailments may be first detected on skin, e.g., purpura from leukemias, nodules from metastases of internal malignancy, hyperpigmentation from Addison's disease, etc.

This book represents a small attempt to bridge the gap or a humble dialogue to communicate. This endeavor, however, has been based totally on visual language, which remains the basic conversation in clinical dermatology. However, this small book would never be able to substitute larger textbooks or atlas published earlier with the same mission and above all practical clinical training and day-to-day practice.

The book would never be written unless the continuous urge, encouragement, and request of Mr Tarun Duneja, the General Manager (Publishing) of M/s Jaypee Brothers Medical Publishers (P) Ltd, New Delhi, India, the eminent medical publisher of the country, who had a long experience and association with our medical fraternity. I must give deep regards to him and his entire publishing team, both in New Delhi and in Kolkata, who have wholeheartedly supported this project.

I must also give sincere thanks to Mr Tapas Kr Kayal, for doing the DTP and all laborious computer jobs for me in spite of his period of personal grief and turmoil.

I feel all my efforts would go in vain unless the readers find the book suitable for their need. Any clarification or queries may be made to me directly by e-mail (drsanjayghosh1@gmail.com).

Sanjay Ghosh

Contents

Case 1 1
Case 2 3
Case 3 5
Case 4 7
Case 5 9
Case 6 11
Case 7 13
Case 8 15
Case 9 17
Case 10 19
Case 11 21
Case 12 23
Case 13 25
Case 14 27
Case 15 29
Case 16 31
Case 17 33
Case 18 35
Case 19 37
Case 20 39
Case 21 41
Case 22 43
Case 23 45
Case 24 47
Case 25 49
Case 26 51
Case 27 53
Case 28 55
Case 29 57
Case 30 59
Case 31 61
Case 32 63
Case 33 65
Case 34 67
Case 35 69

Case	Page
Case 36	71
Case 37	73
Case 38	75
Case 39	77
Case 40	79
Case 41	81
Case 42	83
Case 43	85
Case 44	87
Case 45	89
Case 46	91
Case 47	93
Case 48	95
Case 49	97
Case 50	99
Case 51	101
Case 52	103
Case 53	105
Case 54	107
Case 55	109
Case 56	111
Case 57	113
Case 58	115
Case 59	117
Case 60	119
Case 61	121
Case 62	123
Case 63	125
Case 64	127
Case 65	129
Case 66	131
Case 67	133
Case 68	135
Case 69	137
Case 70	139
Case 71	141
Case 72	143
Case 73	145
Case 74	147
Case 75	149

Contents

Case 76	151
Case 77	153
Case 78	155
Case 79	157
Case 80	159
Case 81	161
Case 82	163
Case 83	165
Case 84	167
Case 85	169
Case 86	171
Case 87	173
Case 88	175
Case 89	177
Case 90	179
Case 91	181
Case 92	183
Case 93	185
Case 94	187
Case 95	189
Case 96	191
Case 97	193
Case 98	195
Case 99	197
Case 100	199
Case 101	201
Case 102	203
Case 103	205
Case 104	207
Case 105	209
Case 106	211
Case 107	213
Case 108	215
Case 109	217
Case 110	219
Case 111	221
Case 112	223
Case 113	225
Case 114	227
Case 115	229

Case 116	231
Case 117	233
Case 118	235
Case 119	237
Case 120	239
Case 121	241
Case 122	243
Case 123	245
Case 124	247
Case 125	249
Case 126	251
Case 127	253
Case 128	255
Case 129	257
Case 130	259
Case 131	261
Case 132	263
Case 133	265
Case 134	267
Case 135	269
Case 136	271
Case 137	273
Case 138	275
Case 139	277
Case 140	279
Case 141	281
Case 142	283
Case 143	285
Case 144	287
Case 145	289
Case 146	291
Case 147	293
Case 148	295
Case 149	297
Case 150	299
Case 151	301
Case 152	303
Case 153	305
Case 154	307
Case 155	309

Case 156	311
Case 157	313
Case 158	315
Case 159	317
Case 160	319
Case 161	321
Case 162	323
Case 163	325
Case 164	327
Case 165	329
Case 166	331
Case 167	333
Case 168	335
Case 169	337
Case 170	339
Case 171	341
Case 172	343
Case 173	345
Case 174	347
Case 175	349
Case 176	351
Case 177	353
Case 178	355
Case 179	357
Case 180	359
Case 181	361
Case 182	363
Case 183	365
Case 184	367
Case 185	369
Case 186	371
Case 187	373
Case 188	375
Case 189	377
Case 190	379
Case 191	381
Case 192	383
Case 193	385
Case 194	387
Case 195	389

Case 196 391
Case 197 393
Case 198 395
Case 199 397
Case 200 399
Case 201 401

Index 403

Case 1

A 35-year-old male had acute-onset grouped painful skin vesicles, some hemorrhagic, on left side of abdomen and loin unilaterally in dermatomal distribution for last 3 days.

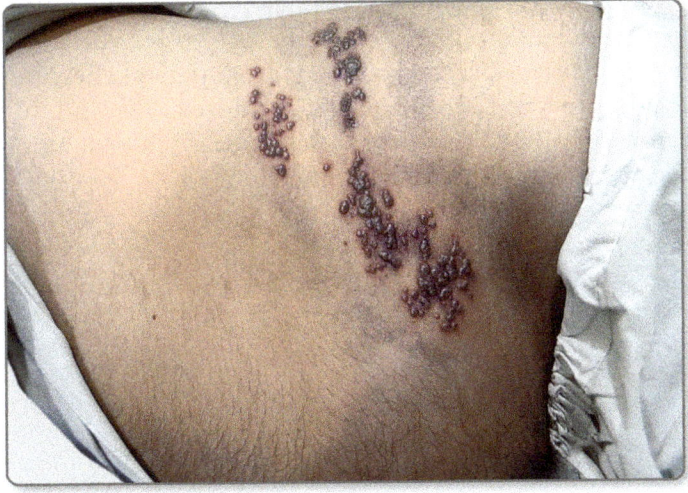

Q. What is the (i) diagnosis, (ii) management and (iii) prevention?

Answers

i. Herpes zoster
ii. Management:
    - Valacyclovir 1,000 mg 8 hourly for 7 days or acyclovir 800 mg 5 times a day for 7 days or famciclovir 500 mg 8 hourly for 7 days
    - Oral antibiotics preferably macrolides for 5–7 days to prevent secondary infection
    - Analgesic and sedatives as per need
iii. *Prevention*: Recombinant nonlive herpes zoster vaccine (injection Shingrix) has been recommended for all persons beyond 50 years of age to prevent herpes zoster. Two doses of 0.5 mL to be given intramuscularly at 2 months apart. However, it should not be during active or convalescence stage of infection.

Case 2

A 56-year-old male had raised skin plaque with web-like extension at the periphery on anterior chest for last about 15 years and complained of excessive itching and pain.

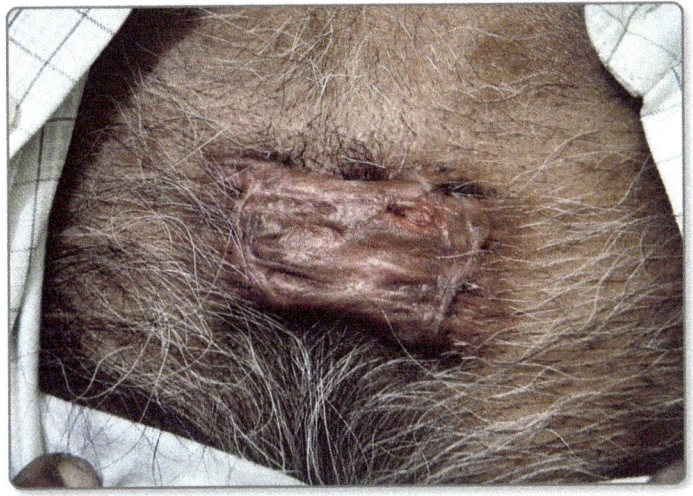

Q. What is the (i) diagnosis and (ii) management?

Answers

i. Keloid
ii. Management:
   - Intralesional triamcinolone injection (dose 10 mg/mL) with or without silicon gel sheet occlusion.
   - Cryotherapy

Case 3

A 29-year-old man had sudden-onset itchy and burning vesicles and papules on right shoulder for last 2 days. The lesions were mostly distributed linearly, but the papulovesicles were neither grouped in arrangement nor limited to dermatomal area.

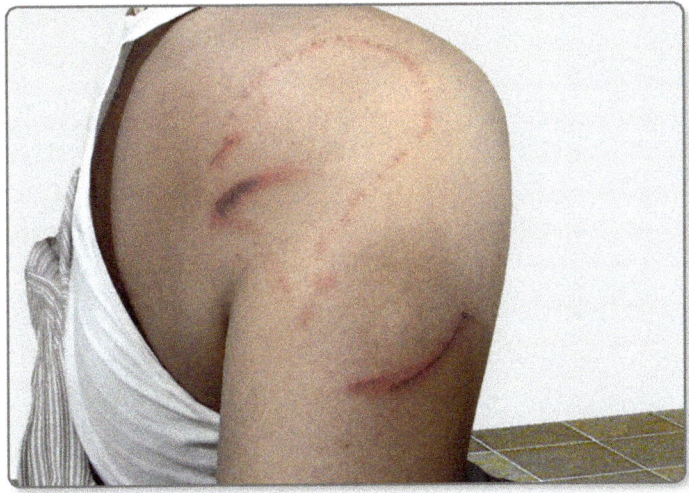

Q. What is the (i) diagnosis and (ii) management?

Answers

i. Insect hypersensitivity
ii. Management:
- Topical potent steroid lotion or cream twice daily for 1 week
- Oral antihistamines
- Oral antibiotics (short course)

Case 4

A 62-year-old lady had developed acute onset pruritic erythematous eruption with papulovesicles and oozing on dorsum of both feet for last 2 weeks after wearing a leather shoe. She had also vesicular eruption on both hands for last 1 week.

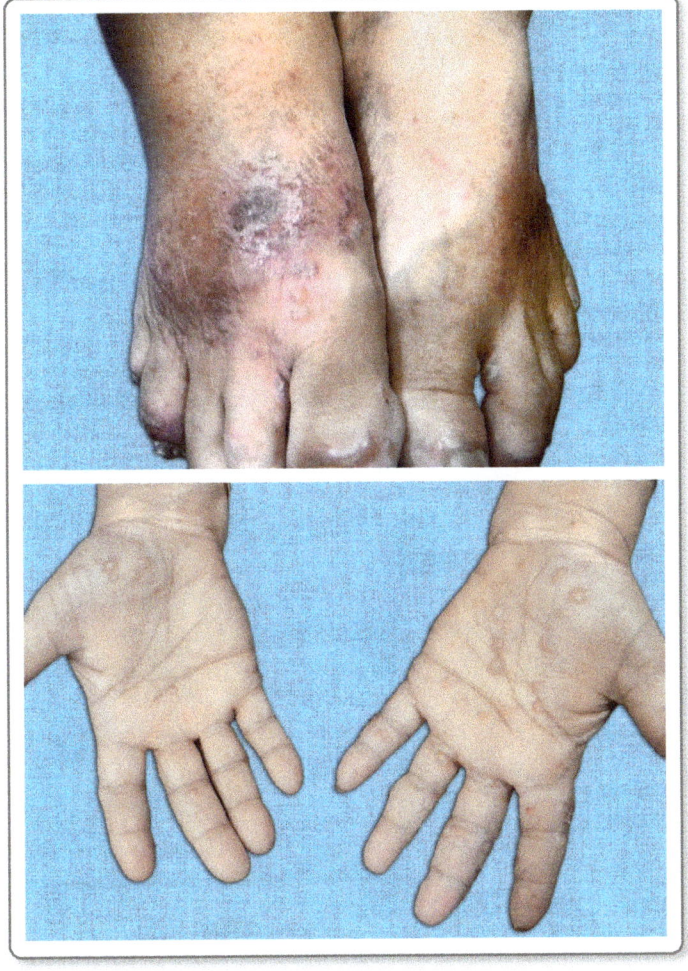

Q. What is the (i) diagnosis and (ii) management?

Answers

i. Acute contact dermatitis (feet) with id eruption (hands) [allergic contact dermatitis (ACD) stage IIIA].
ii. Management:
   - Topical corticosteroid (potent) cream on feet and hands
   - Oral antihistamines
   - Oral antibiotics (short course)
   - Oral corticosteroids (short course), if refractory
   - Allergic patch test to detect nature of footwear allergens

Case 5

A 41-year-old lady had whitish plaque on tongue for last 2 years, which cannot be removed by scraping. She had also reticulated pattern of whitish eruption on her buccal mucosa for same duration.

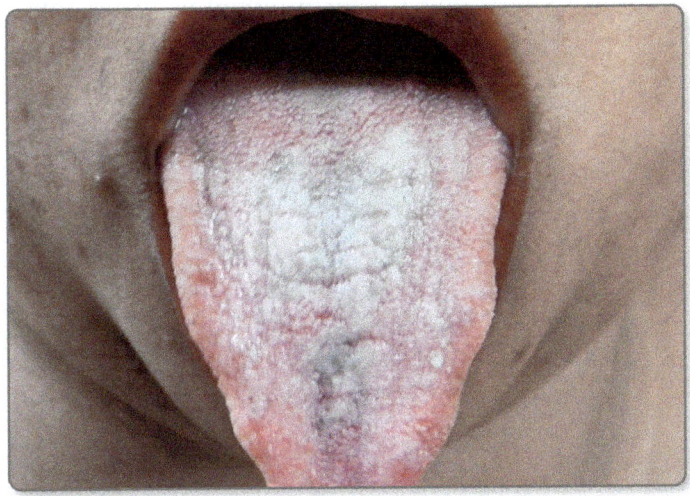

Q. What is the (i) diagnosis and (ii) management?

Answers

i. Oral lichen planus (tongue)
ii. Management:
   - Replacement of metal (including gold) or amalgam dental restorations, if present
   - Topical corticosteroids in orabase followed by topical tacrolimus 0.1% or pimecrolimus 1%
   - Topical (clotrimazole troche or mouth paint) or oral antifungal (fluconazole) to reduce secondary *candida* overgrowth

Case 6

A 57-year-old male had history of nonhealing ulceration on left ankle for last 1 year, and on examination he had anesthesia on left leg and feet along with thickened left lateral popliteal nerve.

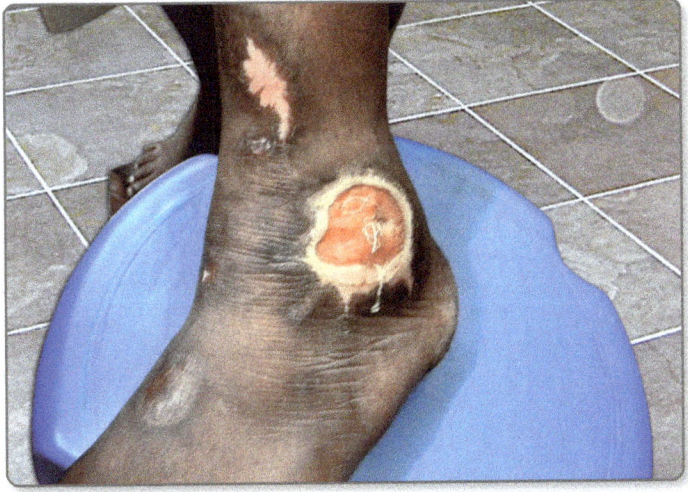

Q. What is the (i) diagnosis and (ii) management?

Answers

i. Leprosy (purely neural) with trophic ulcer
ii. Management:
    - Multidrug therapy [dapsone 100 mg daily, clofazimine 50 mg daily, and rifampicin 600 mg monthly (supervised)].
    - *Care of the ulcer*: Wound swab for bacterial culture and sensitivity, normal saline wash, topical silver sulfadiazine, or fusidic acid cream.
    - *Care of the anesthetic limbs*: Strict avoidance of hot contact and trauma, proper shoe (preferably microcellular rubber).

Case 7

A 33-year-old man developed sudden-onset multiple dark patches upon erythematous background on back and abdomen for last 4 days. He had similar patches on the same sites 8 months back. History revealed that he had taken tinidazole preceding the eruption both the times.

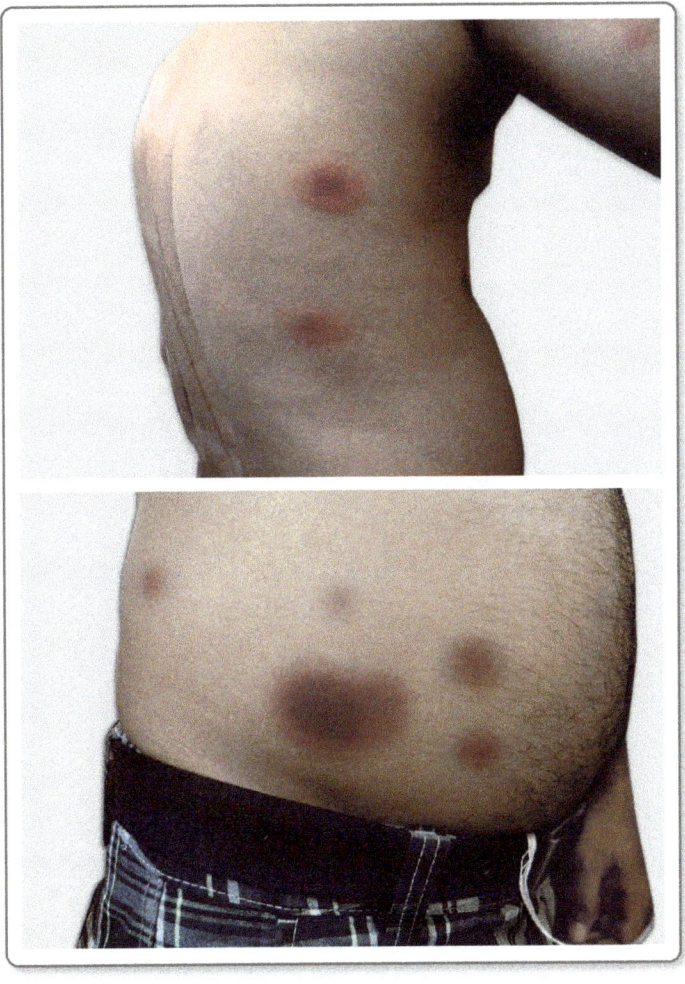

Q. What is the (i) diagnosis and (ii) management?

Answers

i. Fixed drug eruption
ii. Management:
   - Strict avoidance of offending drug and cross-reacting drugs
   - Topical potent steroid once daily for 3 weeks
   - Oral antihistamines

Case 8

A 31-year-lady had localized eczematous eruption on left upper eyelid only for last 2 weeks. She had history of application for last 2 months of a nail polish of new color, which she had not used before.

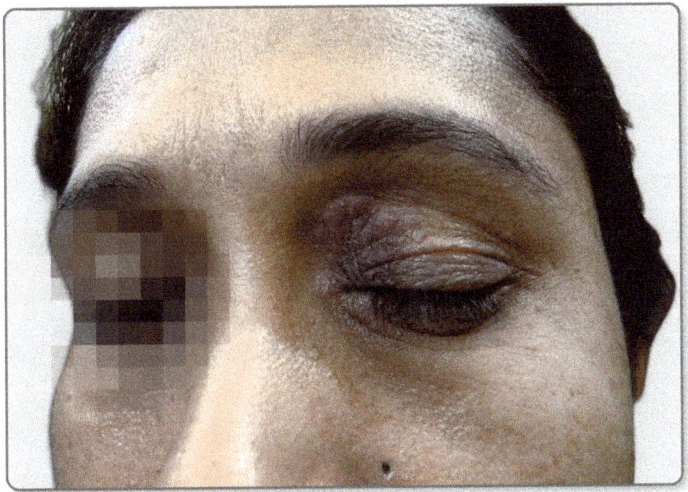

Q. What is the (i) diagnosis and (ii) management?

Answers

i. Allergic contact dermatitis (ACD) (most common site of ACD from nail polish is eyelid, which is usually unilateral)
ii. Management:
   - Strict avoidance of nail polish
   - Low potent steroid cream once daily for 7 days
   - Oral antihistamines for 7 days
   - Allergic patch test to detect nature of allergens

Case 9

An 18-year-old boy had pruritic multiple annular lesions with central clearing and scaly inflamed border with papulovesicles on face, lower abdomen, and groin rapidly spreading for last 2 months.

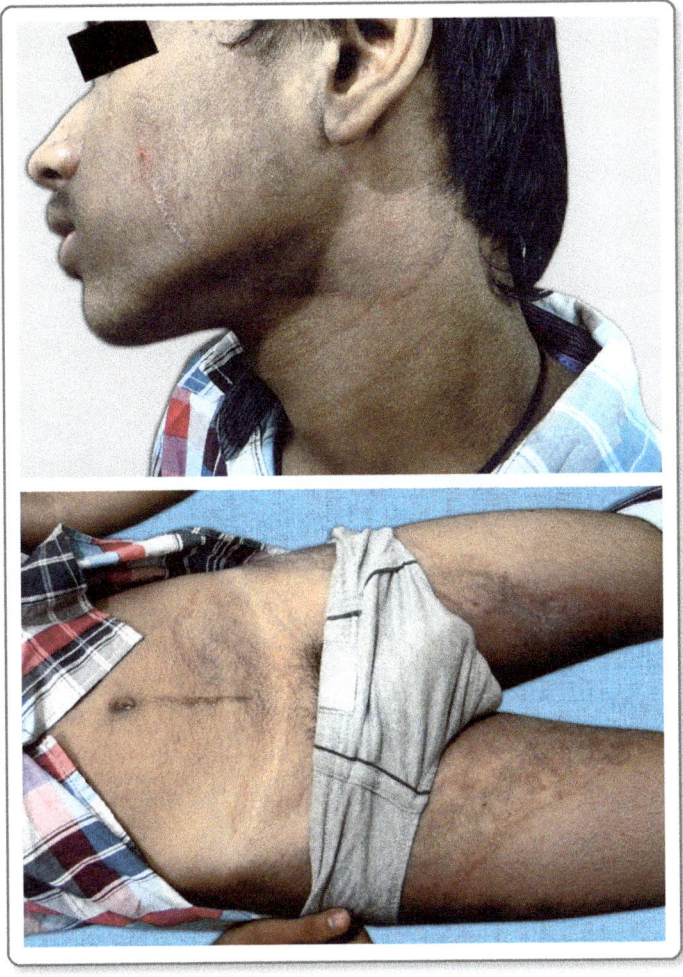

Q. What is the (i) diagnosis and (ii) management?

Answers

i. Tinea faciei and corporis and cruris.
ii. Management:
    - Oral itraconazole 200 mg OD for 14 days
    - Or oral terbinafine 250 mg OD for 14 days
    - Or oral fluconazole 150 mg once/week for 4 weeks
    - Topical, luliconazole, amorolfine, or clotrimazole daily for 4 weeks
    - Maintenance of hygiene (changing/washing/ironing of inner garments, not sharing of clothes, separate washing of clothes, etc.)

Case 10

A 52-year-old lady had chronic eczematous lesions with central ulceration on medial aspect of left ankle for last 4 years. She had associated varicosity of leg veins for last 10 years.

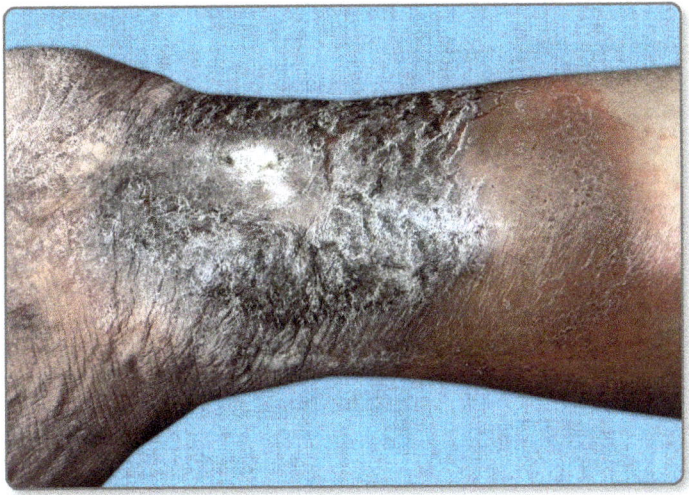

Q. What is the (i) diagnosis and (ii) management?

Answers

i. Stasis dermatitis with ulceration.
ii. Management:
   - Management of varicose veins by stockings, crepe bandage, etc.
   - Avoidance of topical application (higher chance of contact sensitivity)
   - Swab from the wound for bacterial culture and sensitivity
   - Sterile normal saline cleansing
   - Oral antibiotic when needed
   - Oral antihistamines
   - Topical emollient (without paraben, fragrance, and lanolin) on eczematous area

Case 11

A 19-year-old man developed sudden-onset vesicles ("dew-drop on rose petal" like) followed by pustules and crusting on face and upper part of trunk and limb with oral enanthem and history of preceding phase of fever and malaise.

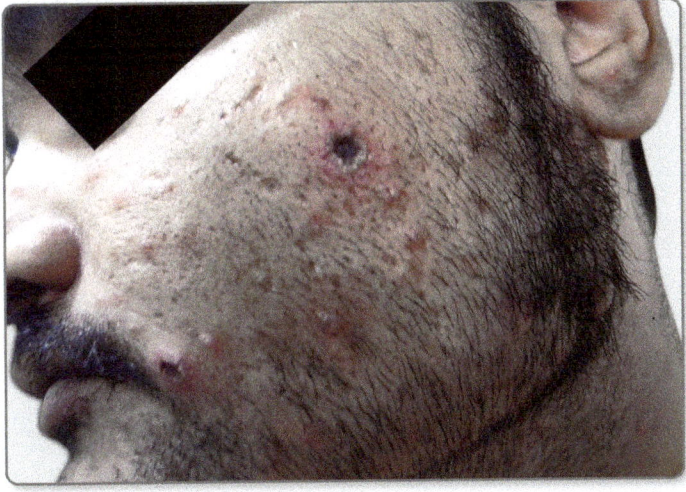

Q. What is the (i) diagnosis and (ii) management?

Answers

i. Varicella (Chickenpox)
ii. Management:
   - Adult varicella is to be always treated by oral antivirals to prevent secondary complications (especially viral pneumonia)
   - Oral valacyclovir 1,000 mg thrice daily for 7 days or acyclovir 800 mg 5 times a day for 7 days or famciclovir 500 mg 8 hourly for 7 days
   - Oral antibiotics preferably macrolides for 5–7 days to prevent secondary infection

Case 12

A 29-year-old male had multiple verrucous lesions on beard area for last 3 months, which are spreading fast. He had history of saloon-shaving before the episode.

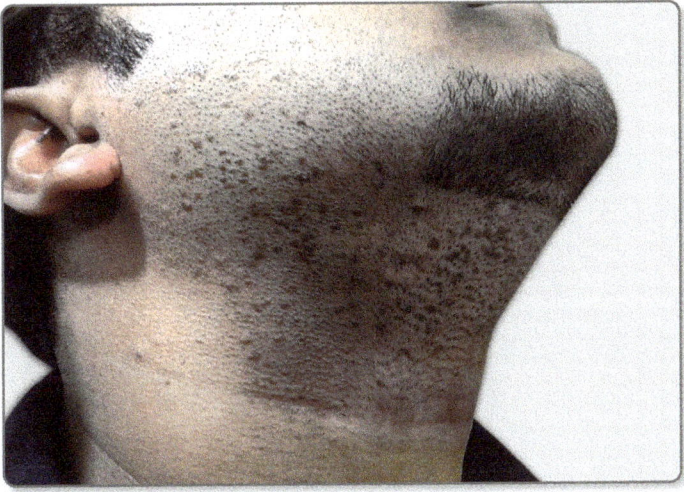

Q. What is the (i) diagnosis and (ii) management?

Answers

i. Verruca plana
ii. Management:
   - Tretinoin 0.05% (keratolytic) to be applied by tooth-pick in the evening for 2–3 hours daily.
   - If delayed response, chemical cautery (by 80% trichloroacetic acid) or light electrocautery should be done by experienced dermatologist.

Case 13

A 34-year-old lady had pigmented circumscribed patch within which more darkly pigmented macular elements on left side of face for last 20 years.

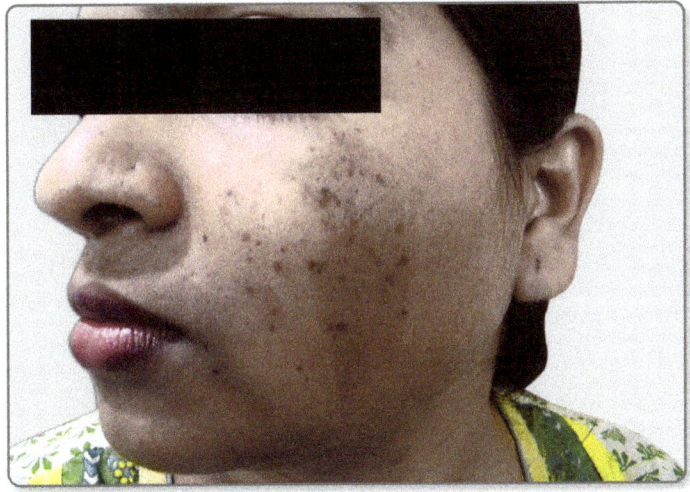

Q. What is the (i) diagnosis and (ii) management?

Answers

i. Nevus spilus
ii. Management:
   - No standard treatment protocol
   - Broad-spectrum sunscreen
   - Cover-mark
   - Atypical new and unstable element within nevus spilus to be histopathologically screened.

Case 14

A 53-year-old female had acneiform lesions with open comedones on face, especially around eyes and temple for last 1 year.

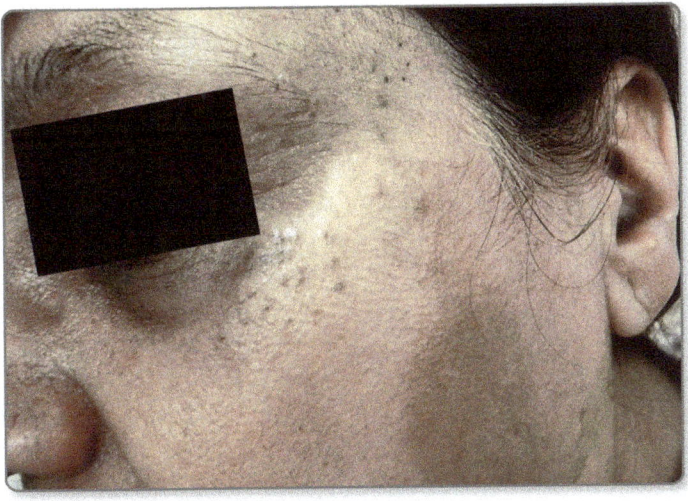

Q. What is the (i) diagnosis and (ii) management?

Answers

i. Senile acne
ii. Management:
   - Tretinoin 0.05% (keratolytic) to be applied by tooth-pick in the evening for 2–3 hours daily.
   - If delayed response, comedones should be removed by comedone extractor.

Case 15

A 24-year-old female had terminal hairs on chin area for last 3 years. She had history of irregular menstruation for last 5 years.

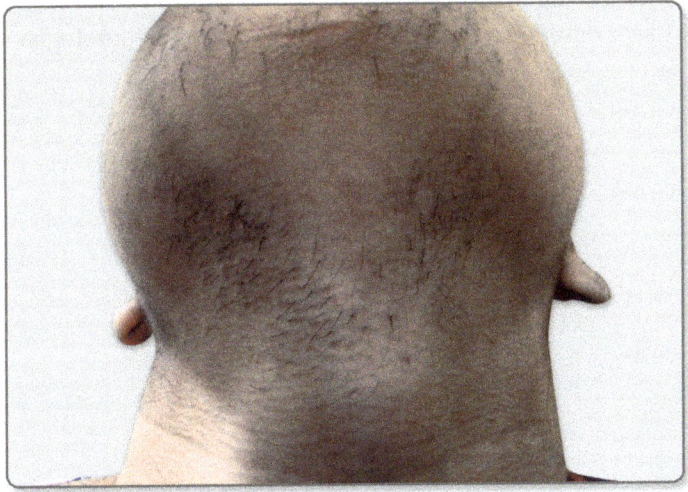

Q. What is the (i) diagnosis and (ii) management?

Answers

i. Hirsutism
ii. Management:
   - Referral to gynecologist/endocrinologist to exclude polycystic ovarian diseases (PCOD), etc., as underlying cause
   - Eflornithine hydrochloride cream twice daily for 3–6 months under monitoring on affected skin
   - Laser or electroepilation by experienced dermatologist

Case 16

A 21-year-old young male had erythematous scaly lesions with crusting bilaterally on face for last 1 year. He had no oral lesions.

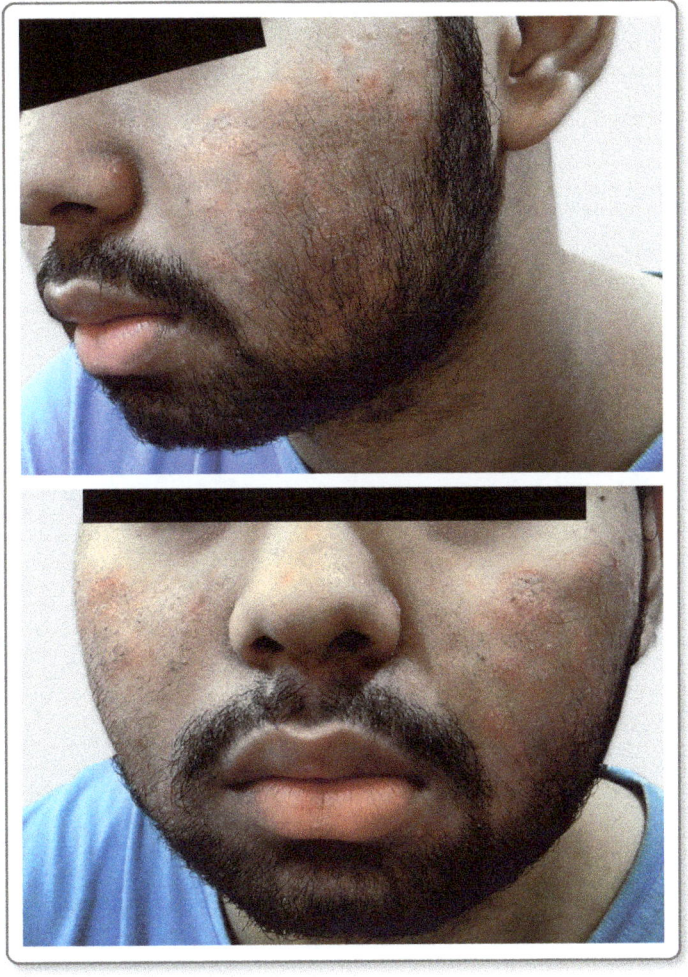

Q. What is the (i) diagnosis and (ii) management?

Answers

i. Pemphigus erythematosus
ii. Management:
    - Referral to dermatologist
    - Skin biopsy to confirm diagnosis
    - To exclude associated LE [by antinuclear antibody (ANA) test]
    - Topical potent steroid
    - High dose of corticosteroids with adjuvant immunosuppressant under experienced dermatologist care

Case 17

A 63-year-old female had acute erythematous eruption on face, forearms, and V-area of neck aggravated by sun exposure, reddish patch around eyelids ("heliotrope erythema") for last 6 months along with proximal myopathy for last 1 month. She had also erythematous papules on knuckles of hands ("Gottron's papules").

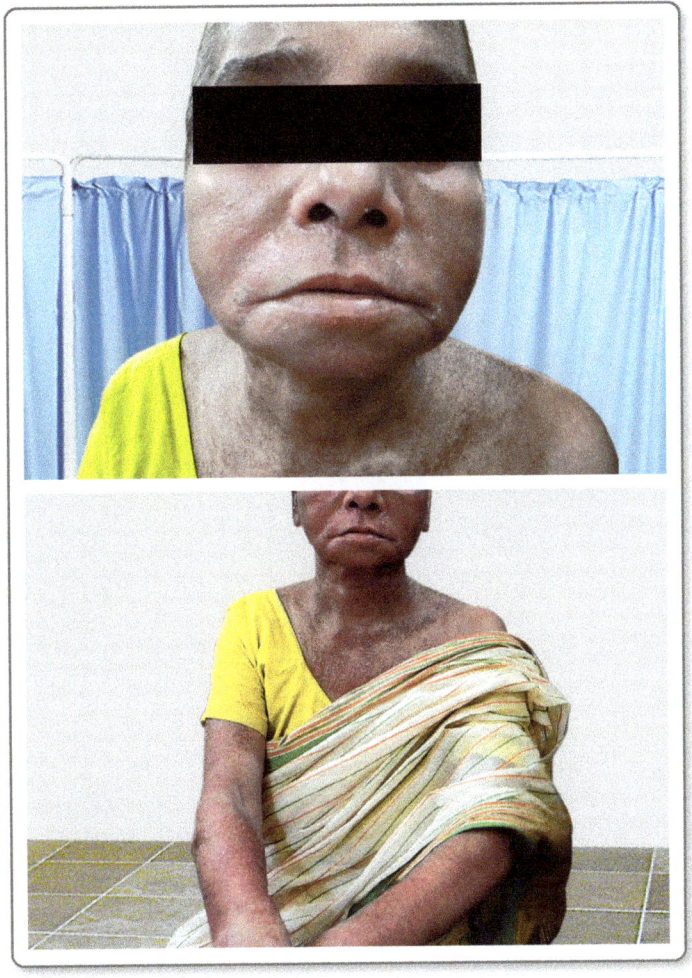

Q. What is the (i) diagnosis and (ii) management?

Answers

i. Dermatomyositis
ii. Management:
   - Referral to dermatologist and rheumatologist
   - Skin biopsy and muscle biopsy to confirm diagnosis
   - To exclude associated systemic lupus erythematosus (SLE)
   - High dose of corticosteroids with adjuvant immunosuppressant under experienced dermatologist and rheumatologist care

Case 18

A 27-year-old male had sudden-onset pruritic erythematous eczematous lesions on both underarms sparing the vault of the axillae (black arrow) for last 1 week. He had history of wearing a new shirt for last 2 weeks.

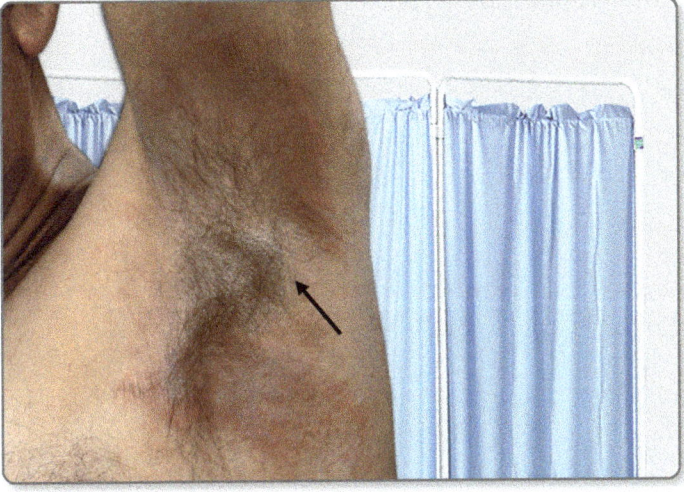

Q. What is the (i) diagnosis and (ii) management?

Answers

i. Allergic contact dermatitis (ACD) from the textiles (in ACD from deodorants vault of the axillae are affected).
ii. Management:
   - Strict avoidance of the offending shirt
   - Mid-potent topical corticosteroids twice daily for 14 days
   - Oral antihistamines for 7 days
   - Allergic patch test to detect relevant allergens

Case 19

A 21-year-old male had hypertrophic lesions on shoulder for 6 months. He had also acneiform eruption on face and trunk or last 4 years.

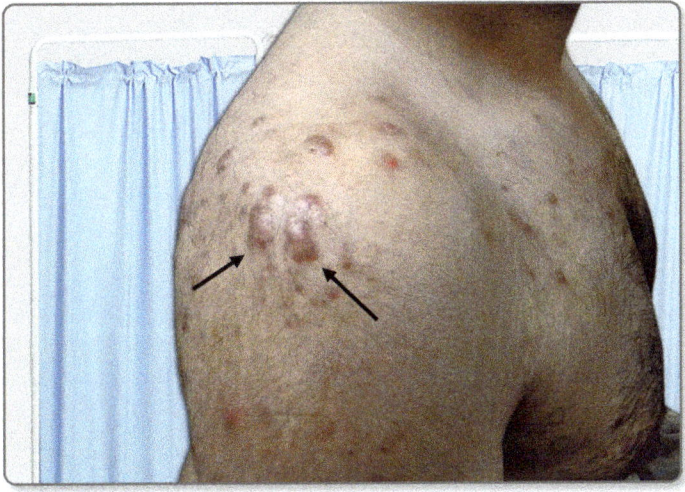

Q. What is the (i) diagnosis and (ii) management?

Answers

i. Acne keloidalis
ii. Management:
   - *Treatment of acne*: Oral isotretinoin, topical benzoyl peroxide
   - Intralesional corticosteroid by expert dermatologist with or without silicon gel sheet application.

Case 20

A 59-year-old male had sudden-onset, painful and tender erythematous plaque on left side of face along with similar two lesions on trunk for last 3 months. The truncal lesions were hypoesthetic. He had faint hypopigmented patches on same sites for last about 2 years.

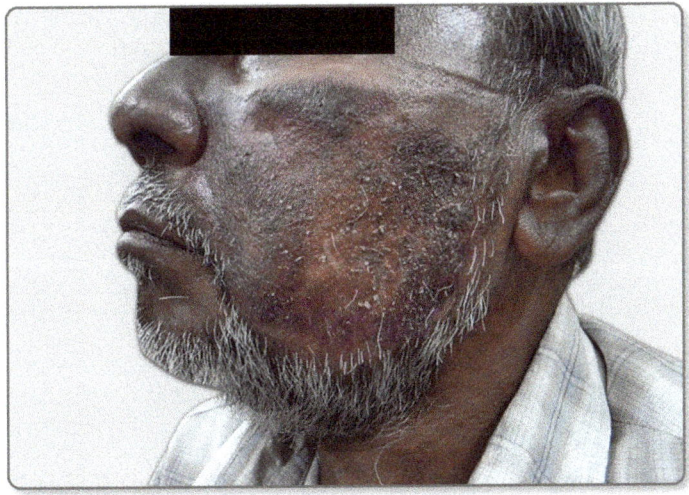

Q. What is the (i) diagnosis and (ii) management?

Answers

i. *Leprosy*: Borderline tuberculoid (BT) with type I reaction.
ii. Management:
   - Multidrug treatment (MDT) consisting of dapsone 100 mg daily, clofazimine 50 mg daily, and rifampicin 600 mg monthly (supervised)
   - Oral prednisolone 60 mg OD to be tapered over 6–8 weeks.

Case 21

A 21-year-old obese male had nonpruritic, velvety thickened skin on neck for last 3 years. He had strong family history of diabetes in both his parents.

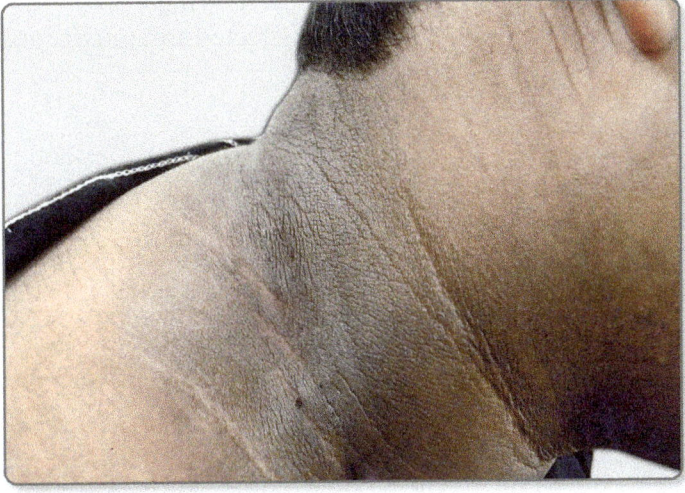

Q. What is the (i) diagnosis and (ii) management?

Answers

i. Acanthosis nigricans
ii. Management:
   - To measure serum insulin level and blood sugar profile
   - Referral to endocrinologist
   - Reduce obesity
   - Regular physical exercise
   - Oral metformin if serum insulin level is high.
   - Topical tretinoin 0.5% cream on affected area once at night gently.

Case 22

A 35-year-old male palmoplantar well-defined scaly plaques (yellow arrow) for last 2 years aggravating in winter with nail pittings. He has also dactylitis (red arrow) and terminal interphalangeal joint involvement and deformity (white arrows).

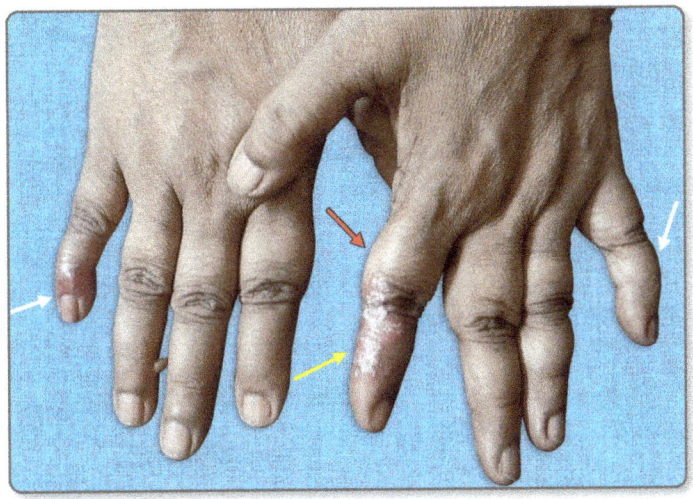

Q. What is the (i) diagnosis and (ii) management?

Answers

i. Psoriasis with psoriatic arthritis (PsA)
ii. Management:
   - Referral to dermatologist and rheumatologist
   - Oral methotrexate/apremilast/biologics under their supervision
   - Topical potent steroid followed by topical calcipotriene locally on skin plaques once daily
   - Topical emollients locally once daily

Case 23

A 41-year-old man, diabetic, had pruritic scaly eruption on both feet, especially involving interdigital areas for last 2 years which used to be aggravated during summer and rainy season.

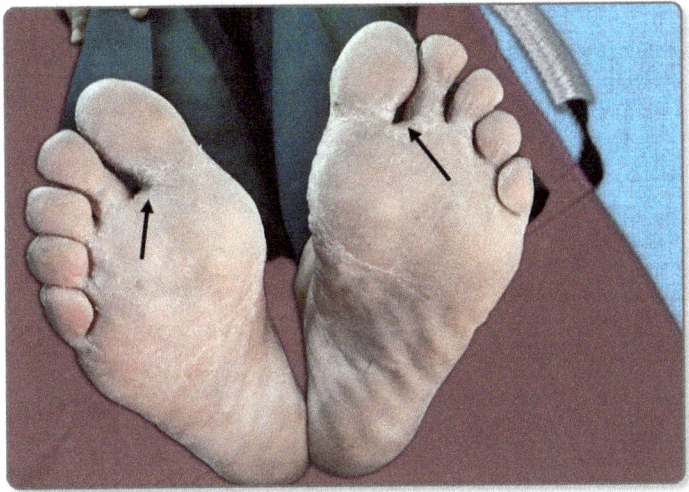

Q. What is the (i) diagnosis and (ii) management?

Answers

i. Tinea pedis
ii. Management:
   - Oral itraconazole 200 mg OD for 14 days
   - Or oral terbinafine 250 mg OD for 14 days
   - Or oral fluconazole 150 mg once/week for 4 weeks
   - Topical, luliconazole, amorolfine, or clotrimazole daily for 4 weeks
   - Maintenance of hygiene (changing/washing/ironing of inner garments, not sharing of clothes, separate washing of clothes, etc.)
   - To keep the feet dry
   - To use cotton socks and airy loose-fitting shoes

Case 24

A 31-year-old man had history of chronic erosive papulovesicular lesions on groins and axillae for last 20 years mostly aggravating during summer and rainy season. He had strong family history of similar diseases in his family. Topical and systemic antifungal treatment did not help him at all.

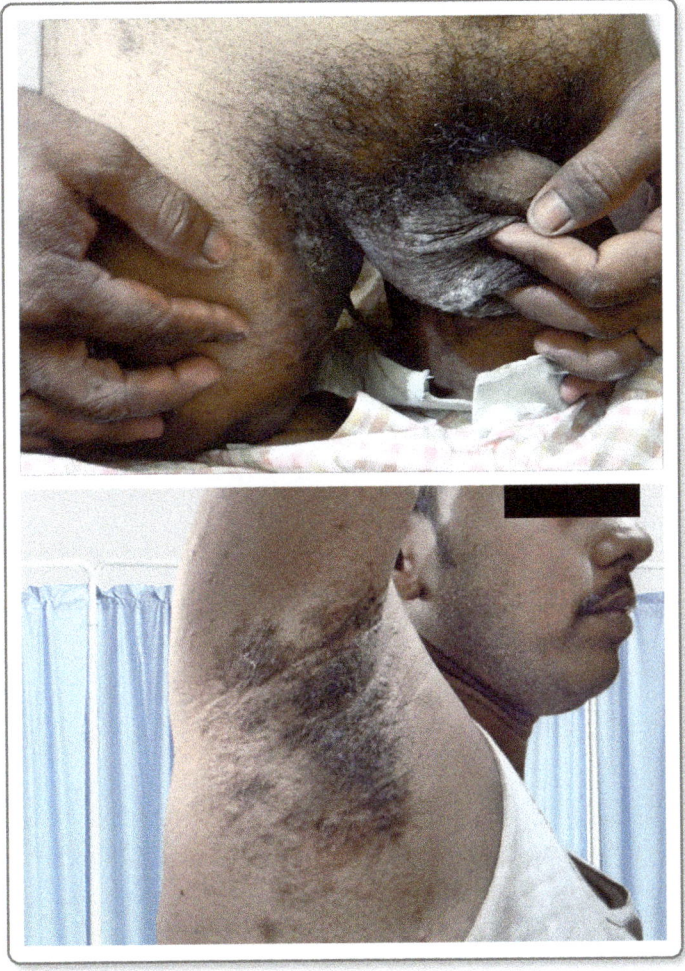

Q. What is the (i) diagnosis and (ii) management?

Answers

i. Hailey–Hailey disease
ii. Management:
   - Minimizing friction and sweating
   - Emollient containing antibacterials
   - Soap substitutes
   - Antiseptic bath additives
   - Moderately potent topical corticosteroids with or without antibacterials and antifungals.

Case 25

A 54-year-old male had chronic pruritic erythematous lichenified (thickening of the skin, increased criss-cross markings of skin looking like "lichen") lesions on both lower legs and dorsum of feet for last 3 years.

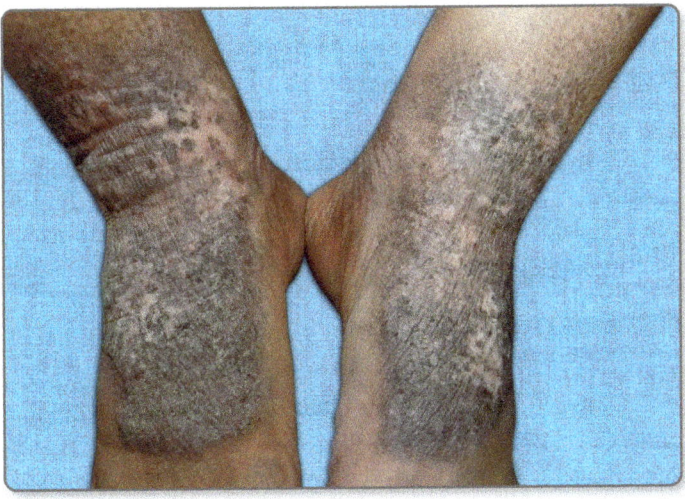

Q. What is the (i) diagnosis and (ii) management?

Answers

i. Lichen simplex chronicus
ii. Management:
   - Topical superpotent topical corticosteroids for 2 weeks followed by low potent corticosteroids for 6 weeks
   - Oral antihistamines (preferably sedative antihistamines)

Case 26

A 14-year-old male had generalized dry "fish-like" scales sparing flexors (black arrow) since infancy which used to aggravate in winter. He had history of similar illness in his father.

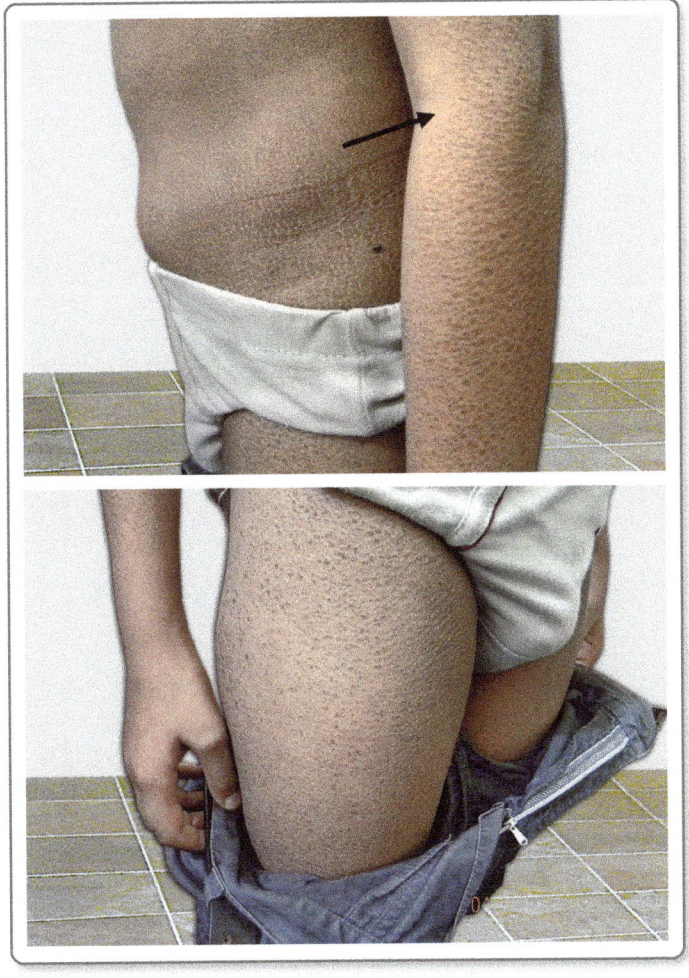

Q. What is the (i) diagnosis and (ii) management?

Answers

i. Ichthyosis vulgaris
ii. Management:
   - Skin hydration by adequate bath followed by immediate application of moisturizer
   - Mild keratolytics like salicylic acid, lactic acid, urea, and propylene glycol application

Case 27

A 31-year-old man had pruritic purpuric eruption for last 4 days. The purpura were palpable. He had history of taking a nonsteroidal anti-inflammatory drug (NSAID) (nimesulide) 1 week back for joint pain.

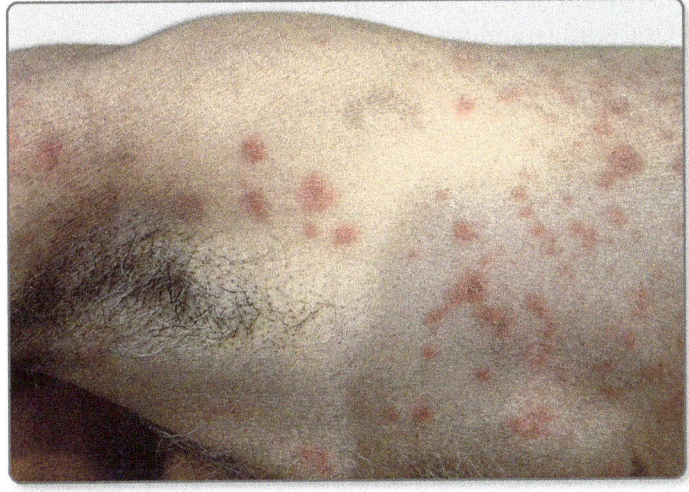

Q. What is the (i) diagnosis and (ii) management?

Answers

i. Allergic purpura
ii. Management:
   - Withdrawal of the offending drug
   - Strict avoidance of the offending drug
   - Urine screening for red blood cell (RBC) to exclude renal involvement
   - Exclusion of systemic involvement
   - Oral antihistamines
   - Topical calamine lotion
   - Topical mid-potent corticosteroid
   - *If refractory*: Oral corticosteroids (short course)

Case 28

A 28-year-old lady had diffuse scarring alopecia for last 6 months. On examination, minute keratotic papules were seen at the hair follicles.

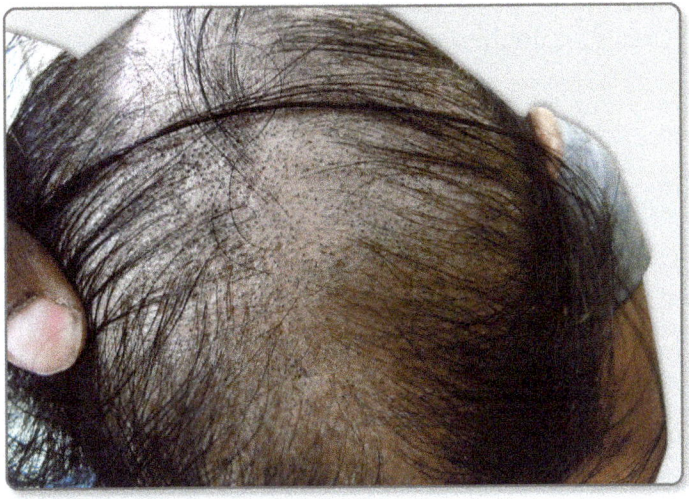

Q. What is the (i) diagnosis and (ii) management?

Answers

i. Lichen planopilaris
ii. Management:
   - Referral to dermatologist
   - Histopathological confirmation of diagnosis
   - High potent topical corticosteroids
   - Systemic corticosteroids (30–40 mg) for 12 weeks
   - Oral isotretinoin under supervision

Case 29

A 54-year-old male had pruritic multiple papular eruption with central keratotic plug (white arrows) predominantly on extensor surface of the limbs for last 3 months. He had been suffering from uncontrolled diabetes.

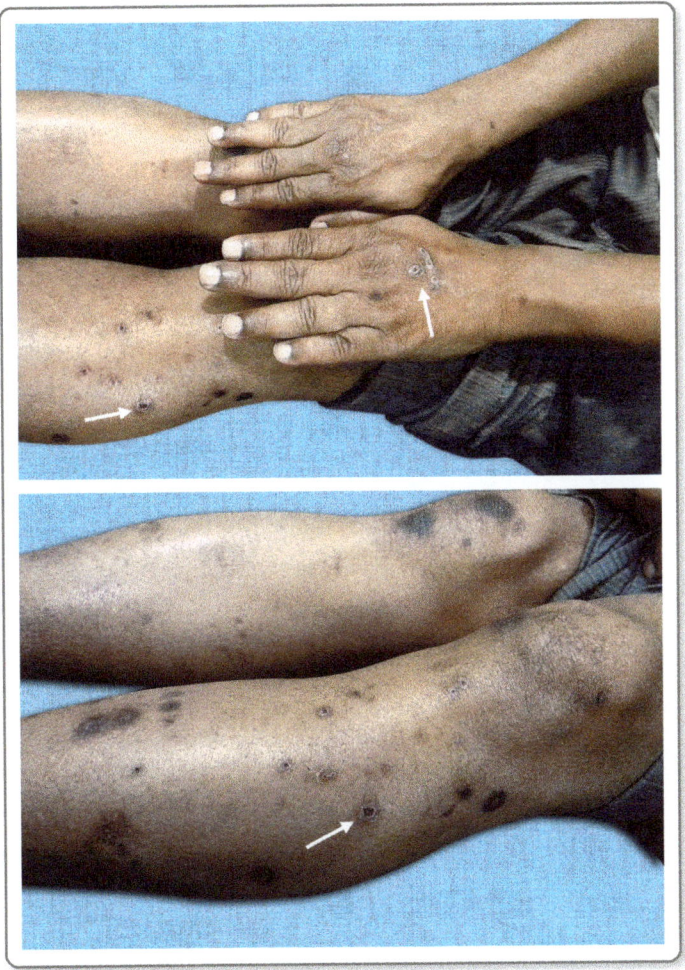

Q. What is the (i) diagnosis and (ii) management?

Answers

i. Perforating folliculitis
ii. Management:
   - Referral to endocrinologists to control diabetes
   - Topical tretinoin 0.025% (gradually increased to 0.05%) to apply in the evening
   - PUVA by expert dermatologist

Case 30

A 49-year-old female had an asymptomatic localized hyperpigmented plaque on front of the right side of the chest. On examination, sclerosis was found in the whole lesion.

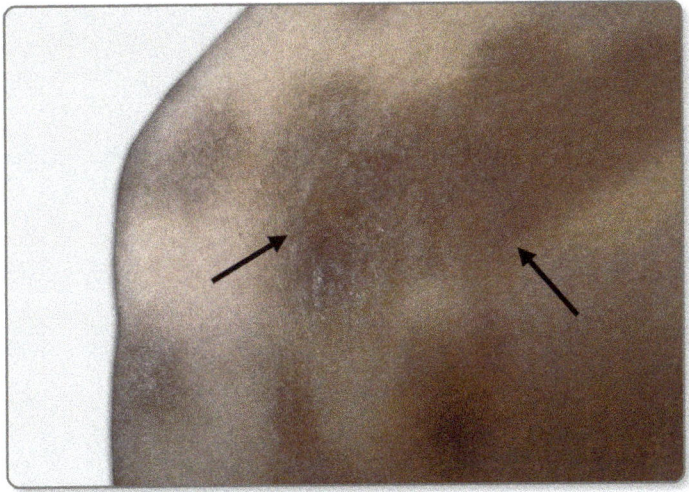

Q. What is the (i) diagnosis and (ii) management?

Answers

i. Morphea (localized scleroderma)
ii. Management:
   - Referral to dermatologist
   - Topical or intralesional corticosteroids
   - Topical calcipotriol

Case 31

A 58-year-old male had sudden development of asymptomatic depigmented lesions on forehead and other part of face for last 6 weeks. On examination, some confetti macules (black arrows) were seen adjacent to the lesions. He had history of application of hair dye containing para-phenylenediamine (PPD) for last 6 months.

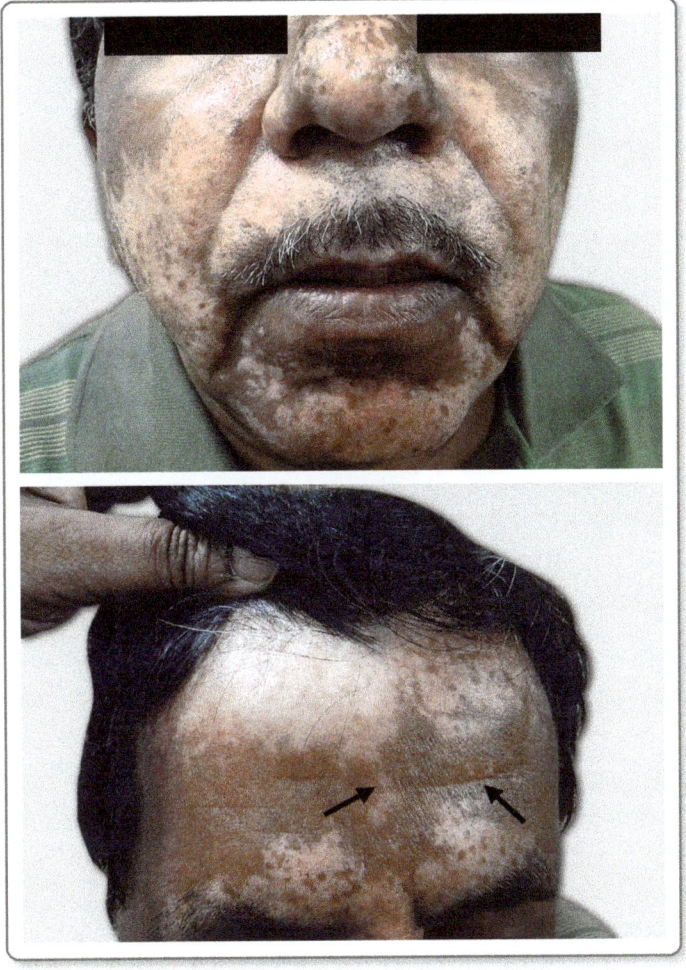

Q. What is the (i) diagnosis and (ii) management?

Answers

i. Chemical vitiligo
ii. Management:
   - Strict avoidance of dye containing PPD
   - Topical mid-potent steroid once daily or topical tacrolimus 0.1% or topical pimecrolimus twice daily
   - If refractory, ultraviolet B (UVB) narrow band or PUVA or PUVAsol or excimer light or laser under expert dermatologist

Case 32

A 29-year-old female had multiple, discrete, tiny, glistening, flesh-colored smooth and flat, round papules on arms and neck for last 3 months.

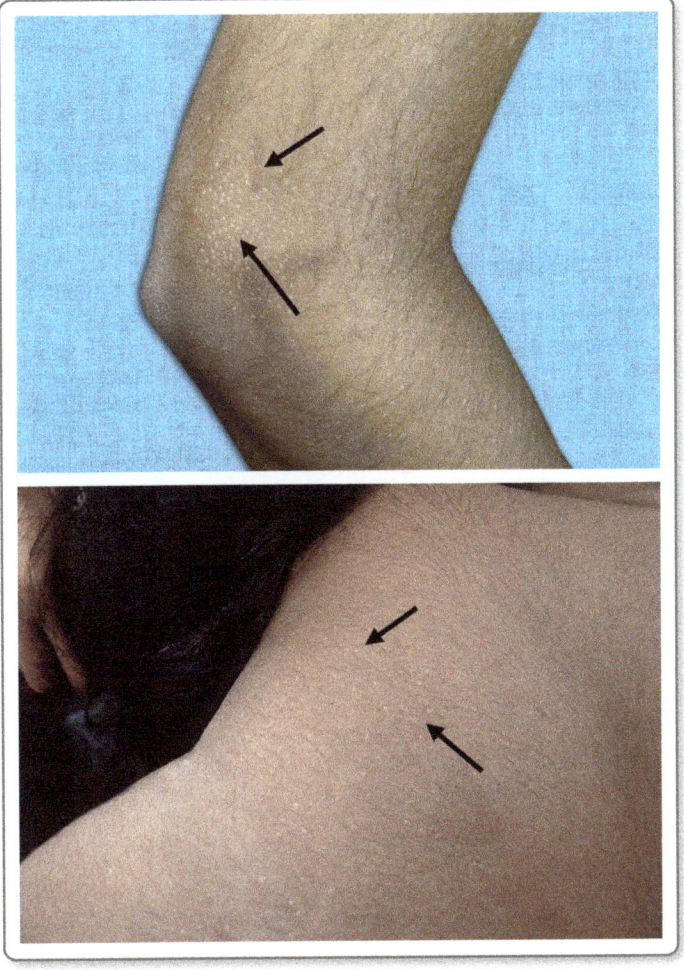

Q. What is the (i) diagnosis and (ii) management?

Answers

i. Lichen nitidus
ii. Management:
   - Topical mid-potent corticosteroid
   - Oral antihistamines (if pruritus)
   - If on sun-exposed area, broad-spectrum sunscreen

Case 33

A 24-year-old young lady had a linear hyperpigmented asymptomatic mark in geometric shape on dorsum of left hand for about last 10 days. Her parents gave the history of her marriage negotiation, which she did not approve. On repeated investigations, she confessed that she has produced the lesion by application of bathroom-cleansing acid.

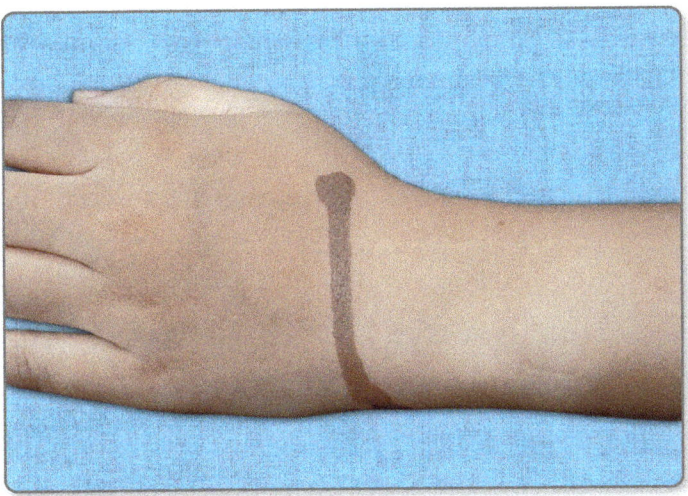

Q. What is the (i) diagnosis and (ii) management?

Answers

i. Dermatitis artefacta
ii. Management:
    - A supportive, nonconfrontational, empathic approach
    - Referral to psychiatrist
    - Mid-potent topical corticosteroid once daily
    - Daytime sunscreen

Case 34

A 31-year-old lady had persistent facial erythema, flushing along with papules and pustules predominantly on convex area for last 3 years.

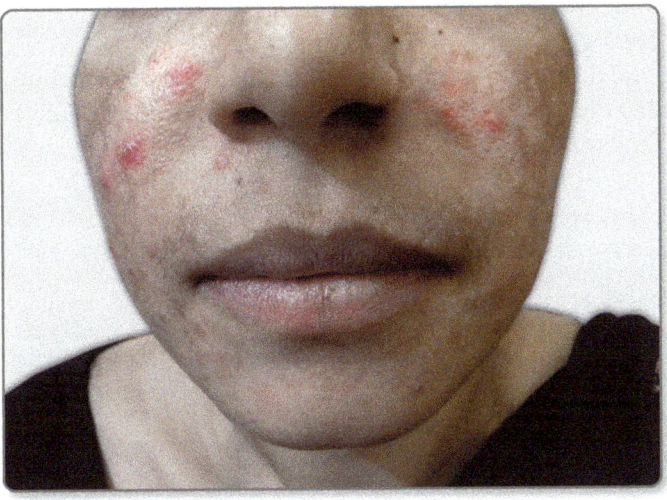

Q. What is the (i) diagnosis and (ii) management?

Answers

i. Rosacea
ii. Management:
   - Topical metronidazole 1% gel twice daily or azelaic acid 15% once daily
   - Topical benzoyl peroxide gel or wash, clindamycin gel or pimecrolimus cream or tacrolimus ointment
   - Topical ivermectin 1% cream
   - Oral doxycycline (low dose: 40 mg daily) or tetracycline (low dose: 250 mg BD) or isotretinoin (low dose: 10–40 mg daily)
   - Oral macrolides or metronidazole

Case 35

A 19-year-old young man had asymptomatic linear atrophic lesion on left axilla for last 3 months. He had history of application of topical steroid and antifungal combination for last 6 months intermittently for itching and rash on axillae.

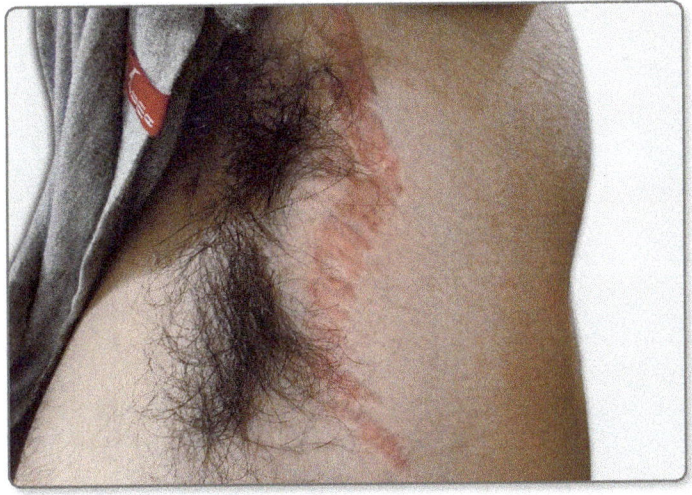

Q. What is the (i) diagnosis and (ii) management?

Answers

i. Striae (steroid-induced)
ii. Management:
   - Strictly avoidance of topical steroid preparation
   - Topical tretinoin 0.025% (gradually increased to 0.05%) daily in evening gently

Case 36

A 27-year-old lady had thick, hyperkeratotic lesions on feet for last 1 year. On examination, the lesions were more tender on lateral pressure than ventral pressure.

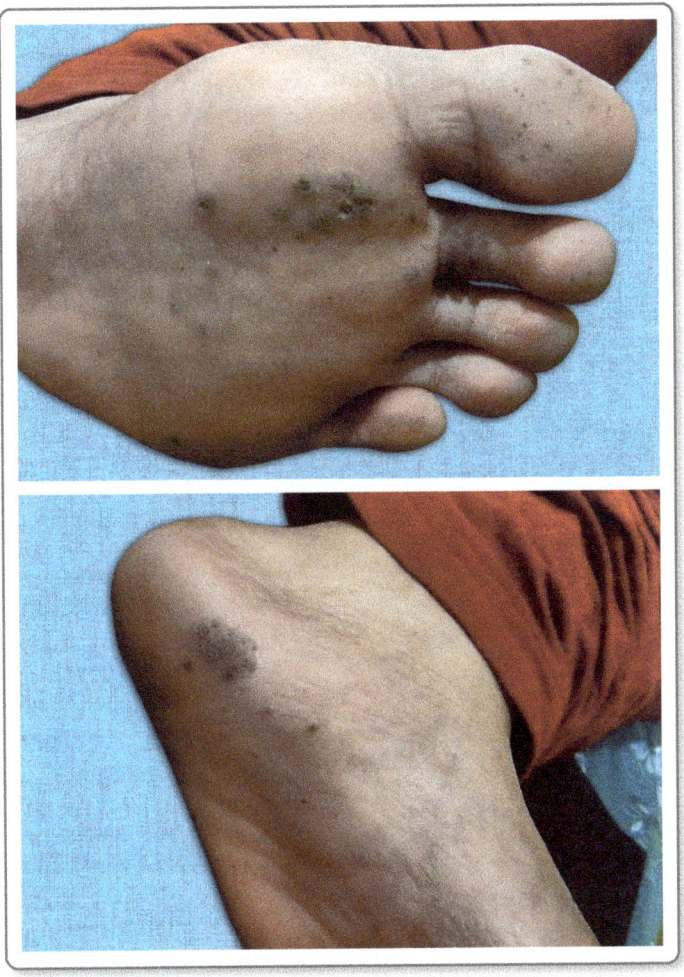

Q. What is the (i) diagnosis and (ii) management?

Answers

i. Plantar verruca
ii. Management:
   - Salicylic acid 16.5%
     - Lactic acid 16.5%
     - Flexible collodion 10 mL Mft pig.
     - To apply on the warts with applicator for 2–3 hours (later overnight)
   - Topical antibacterial once a day
   - If refractory, chemical cautery (by 80% trichloroacetic acid), electrocautery or cryosurgery by trained dermatologist.

Case 37

A 36-year-old lady had gradually developing alopecia in parting region for last 1 year. Her frontal and temporal hair margins are well preserved.

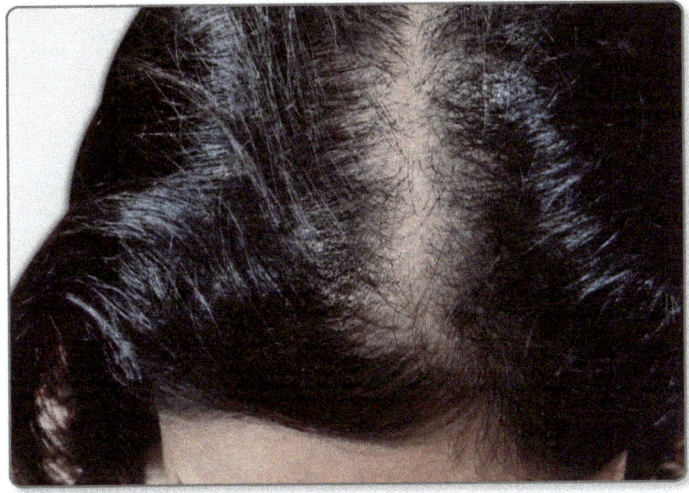

Q. What is the (i) diagnosis and (ii) management?

Answers

i. Female pattern hair loss (Olssen type)
ii. Management:
   - Screening for hematological, gynecological and endocrinological status
   - Topical minoxidil 2% lotion 1 mL twice daily for 6 months.

Case 38

A 57-year-old man had gradually developing alopecia predominantly involving temporal area for last 5 years.

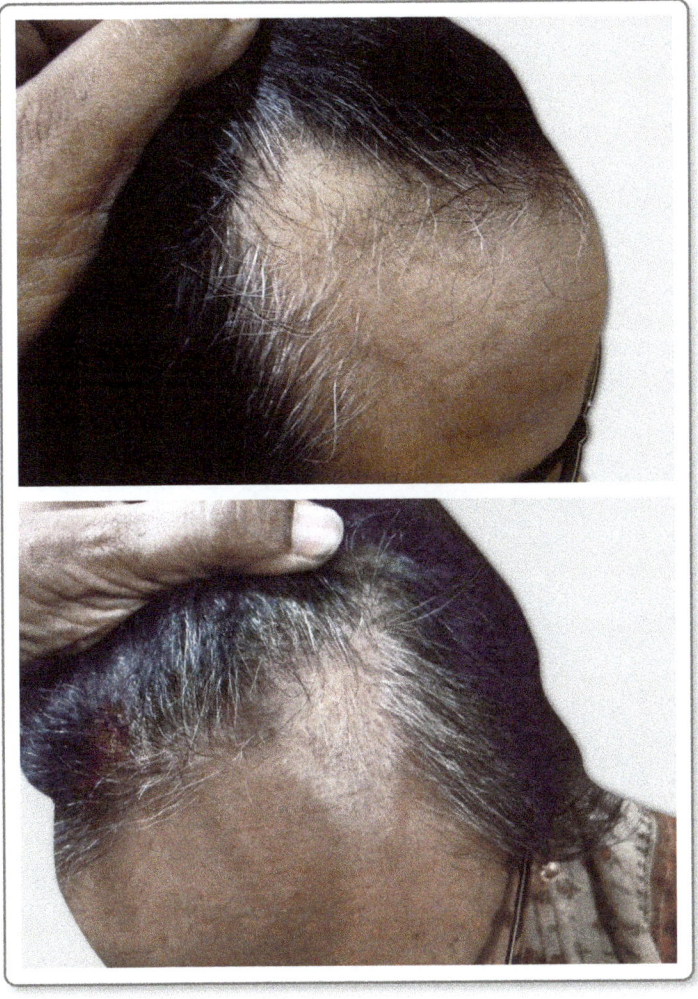

Q. What is the (i) diagnosis and (ii) management?

Answers

i. Male pattern hair loss (MPHL) or AGA (Hamilton–Norwood type)
ii. Management:
   - Topical minoxidil 5% lotion 1 mL twice daily for 6 months
   - Oral finasteride 1 mg daily under supervision of expert dermatologist

Case 39

A 23-year-old young lady had asymptomatic dark-colored papules on face for last 5 years. She had similar lesions in her mother and maternal aunt.

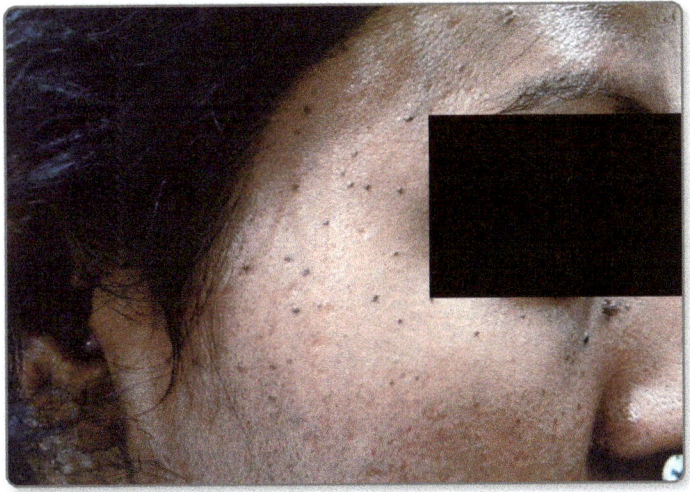

Q. What is the (i) diagnosis and (ii) management?

Answers

i. Dermatosis papulosa nigra
ii. Management:
    - Apply topical tretinoin 0.5% cream in the evening daily with tooth-pick for 3 months.
    - If refractory, light electrofulguration under experienced dermatologist
    - Recurrence frequent

Case 40

A 27-year-old male had severe inflammatory papulopustules and nodules on face with massive scarring and hyperpigmentation for last 8 years.

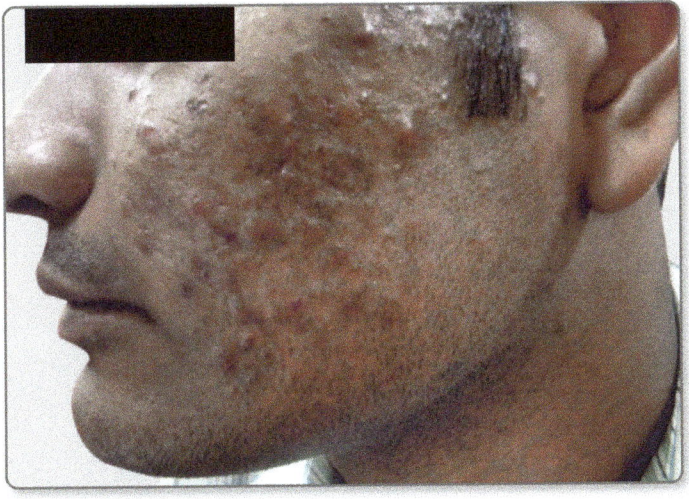

Q. What is the (i) diagnosis and (ii) management?

Answers

i. Acne nodularis
ii. Management:
   - Oral isotretinoin 20 mg twice daily by pretherapy screening and pretherapy monitoring for lipid and liver enzymes level for 3-6 months
   - Topical clindamycin twice daily for 2 months
   - Topical benzoyl peroxide 2.5% gel daily once daily for 6 months
   - After completion of acne treatment, scar management

Case 41

A 25-year-old male had extensive acneiform eruption (black arrows) on arms, back, and chest for last 1 year. The lesions had no comedone and he had no acneiform lesions on face. He had history of application of topical steroid on and off during last 3 years.

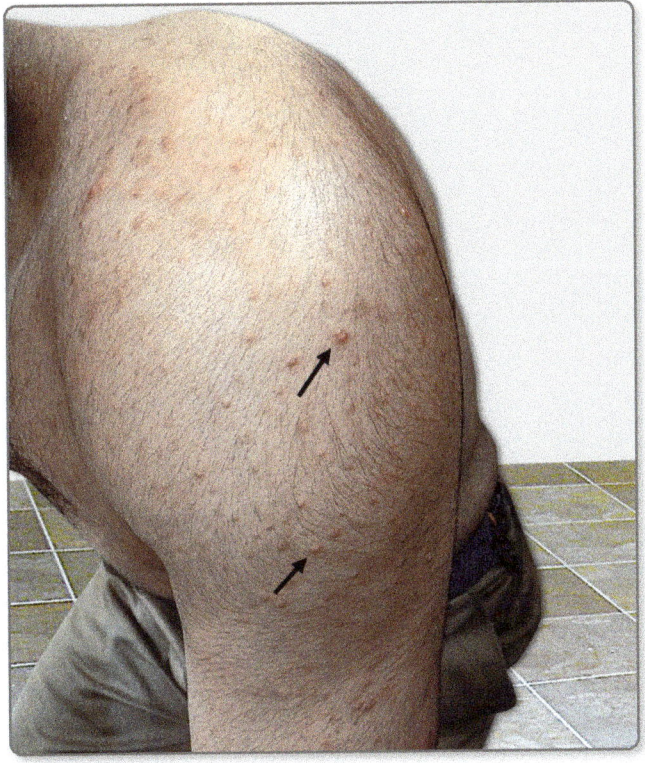

Q. What is the (i) diagnosis and (ii) management?

Answers

i. Steroid acne or folliculitis
ii. Management:
    - Strict avoidance of topical steroid
    - Topical benzoyl peroxide 2.5% gel to apply in the evening daily for 3 months
    - Oral doxycycline, if refractory

Case 42

A 59-year-old male had asymptomatic thick velvety hyperpigmented lesion on forehead and side of face for last 5 years. He had been suffering from diabetes for last 3 years.

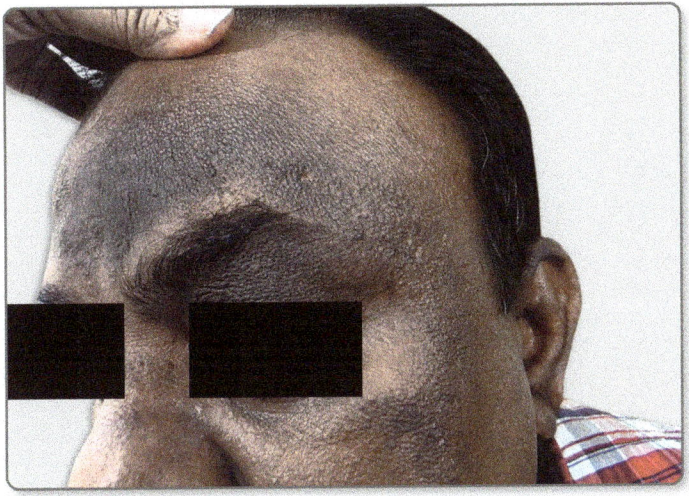

Q. What is the (i) diagnosis and (ii) management?

Answers

i. Acanthosis nigricans
ii. Management:
- Control of diabetes
- Apply topical tretinoin 0.5% cream gently in the evening daily for 3 months.

Case 43

A 41-year-old male had history of bluish appearance of toes and fingers on exposure of cold for last 10 years and tightening (sclerosis) (black arrow) of facial and acral skin for last 3 years. The tip of her digits had become narrow (white arrows).

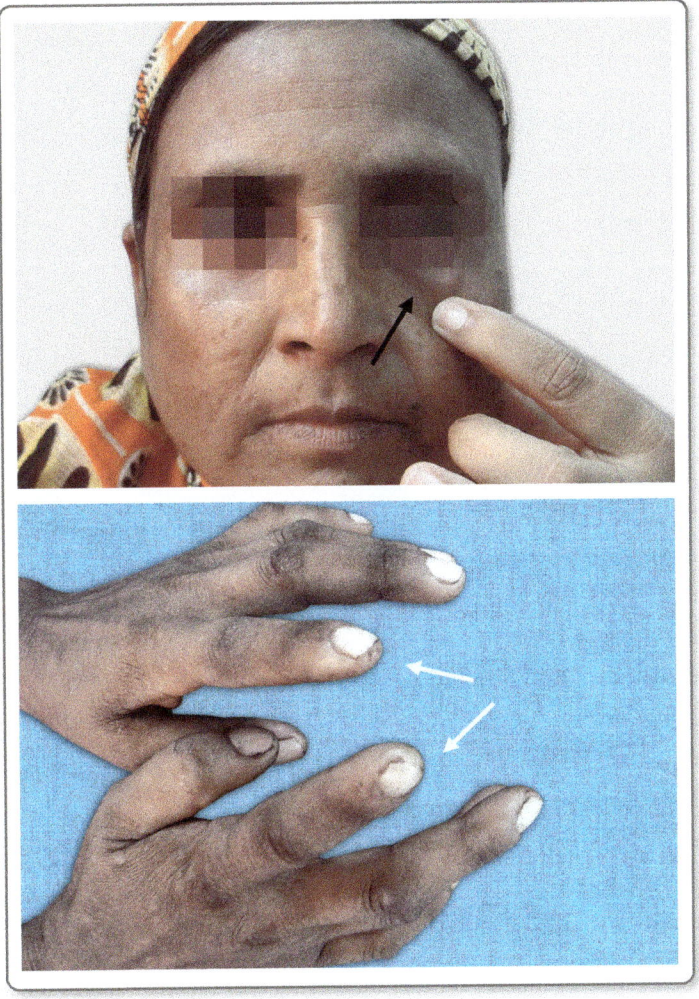

Q. What is the (i) diagnosis and (ii) management?

Answers

i. Systemic scleroderma (limited) [lcSsc]
ii. Management:
   - Referral to dermatologist and rheumatologist
   - Avoidance of cold exposure (to use woolen gloves, socks, etc.)
   - To monitor systemic involvement especially renal and pulmonary organs.

Case 44

A 9-year-old girl had small superficial vesicles (white arrow) on face for last 10 days. The vesicles ruptured to form superficial erosions with yellowish-brown crust (black arrow).

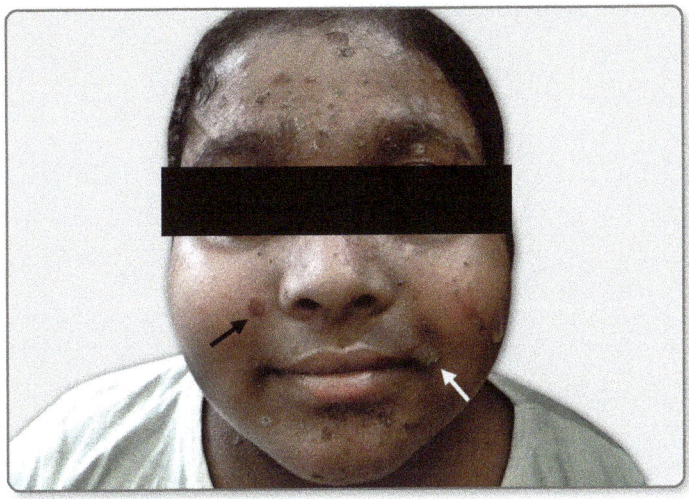

Q. What is the (i) diagnosis and (ii) management?

Answers

i. Impetigo vulgaris
ii. Management:
   - Topical retapamulin or mupirocin or fusidic acid
   - Oral cloxacillin, cephalexin, or erythromycin
   - To watch for nephropathy in later weeks (beta-hemolytic *Streptococcus*, frequent cause of impetigo, may induce glomerulonephritis in certain cases)

Case 45

A 32-year-old male had dark-colored papules (white arrows) on his scrotum for last 10 years with history of occasional hemorrhage (seen on his underclothes as blood-stain). His father had similar problem.

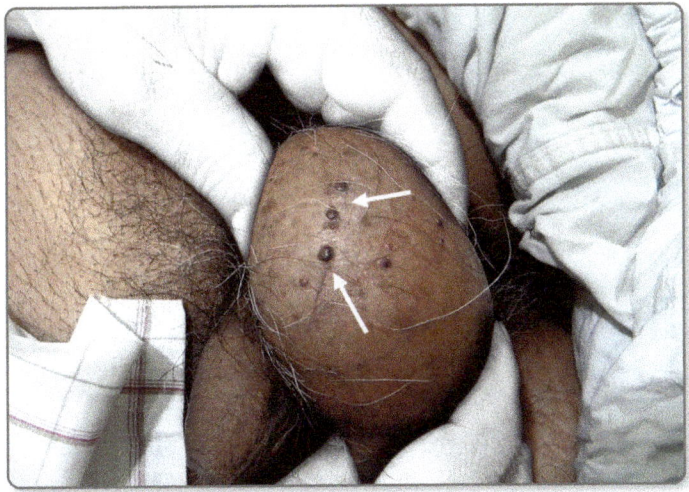

Q. What is the (i) diagnosis and (ii) management?

Answers

i. Angiokeratoma scroti
ii. Management:
   - Referral to dermatologist
   - Light electrofulguration or cryotherapy.

Case 46

A 34-year-old male had acute pruritic erythematous wheals (black arrow) on face and different parts of the body and limbs for last 3 days. He had no history of associated breathing difficulty and choking throat. He had taken food in a restaurant 4 days back.

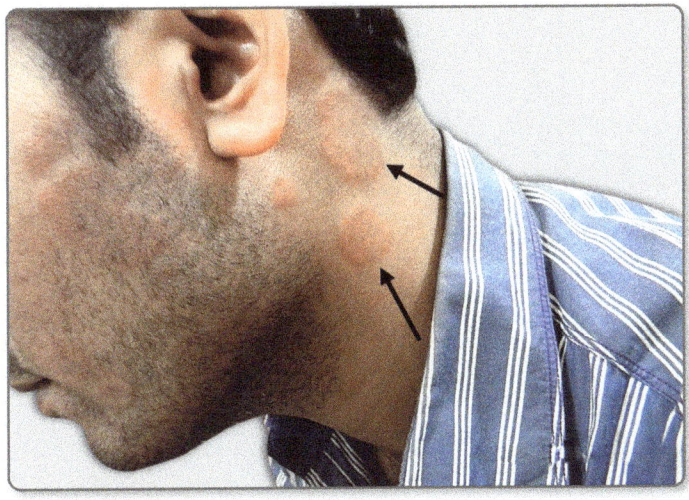

Q. What is the (i) diagnosis and (ii) management?

Answers

i. Acute urticaria (probably due to food-additives)
ii. Management:
   - Strict avoidance of outside food and NSAIDs
   - To watch for acute respiratory symptoms (then immediate emergency hospitalization)
   - Oral antihistamines (if not responding, dose escalation)
   - Short course of systemic steroid, if refractory

Case 47

A 53-year-old male had recurrent oral (black arrow) and genital ulceration for last 5 years. Pathergy test by intradermal normal saline produced positive result (white arrow).

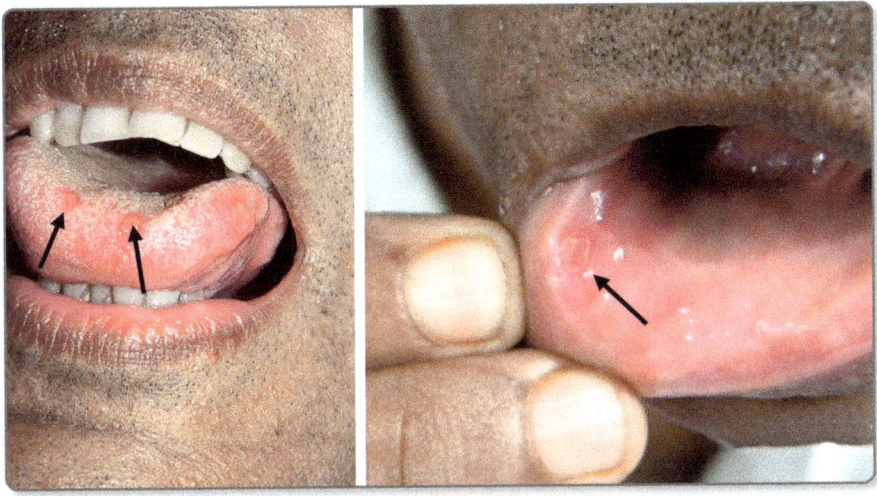

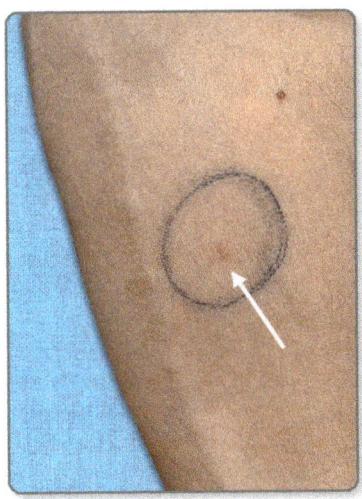

Q. What is the (i) diagnosis and (ii) management?

Answers

i. Behçet's disease
ii. Management:
    - Referral to dermatologist and rheumatologist (to exclude systemic organ involvement especially large vessels and central nervous system)
    - Topical chlorhexidine mouthwash, topical corticosteroids, topical sucralfate
    - Oral tetracycline suspension
    - Oral colchicine or dapsone (under experienced dermatologist).

Case 48

A 45-year-old male, farmer by profession, had pruritic papulovesicular eruption on face, trunk, and limbs for last 2 years mostly aggravated during rainy season. His submental area (white arrow) were spared. He had history of exposure to parthenium plants during his occupation.

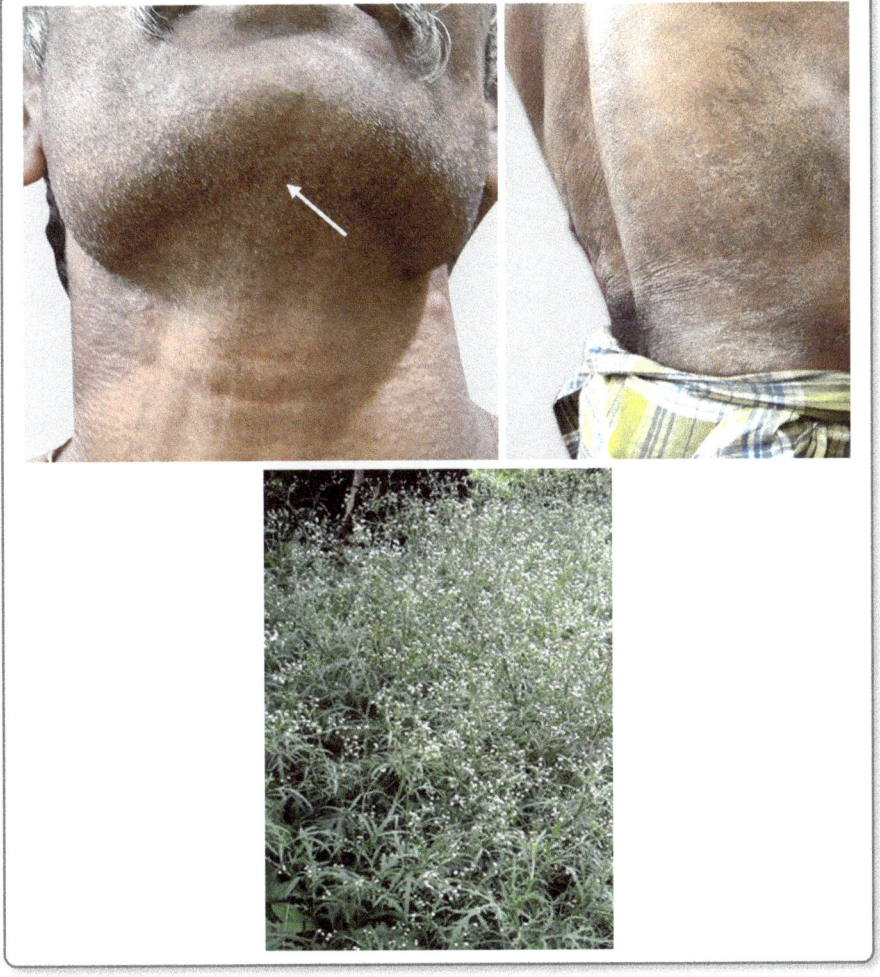

Q. What is the (i) diagnosis and (ii) management?

Answers

i. Photoallergic contact dermatitis (PACD) to parthenium (in airborne contact dermatitis or ABCD submental and retroauricular area are spared).

ii. Management:
- To avoid parthenium and sun exposure as far as possible by using full sleeves, etc.
- Topical low potent steroid or tacrolimus on face
- Topical potent steroid on trunk and limbs
- Antihistamines
- Oral short course steroid, if refractory

Case 49

A 54-year-old female had pruritic violaceous flat-topped papules (white arrows) on thighs, legs, dorsum of feet for last 1 year. On examination, her buccal mucosa showed lacy pattern of whitish plaque (black arrow).

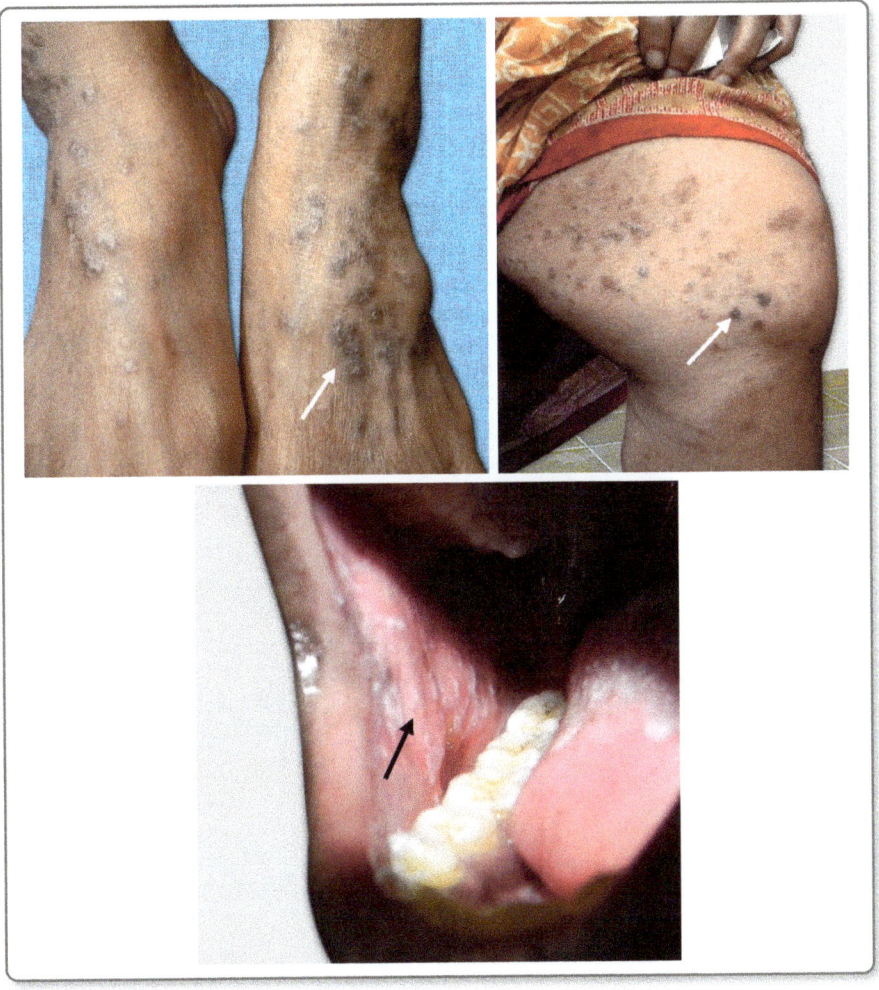

Q. What is the (i) diagnosis and (ii) management?

Answers

i. Lichen planus
ii. Management:
- To avoid oral dental metal fitting, amalgam, if any
- Topical potent steroid on trunk and limbs
- Antihistamines
- Oral short course steroid, if refractory

Case 50

A 43-year-old female had nodular swelling on lower leg (posterior) for last 2 years. Her Mantoux test (5 TU) produced strong positive (18+) result.

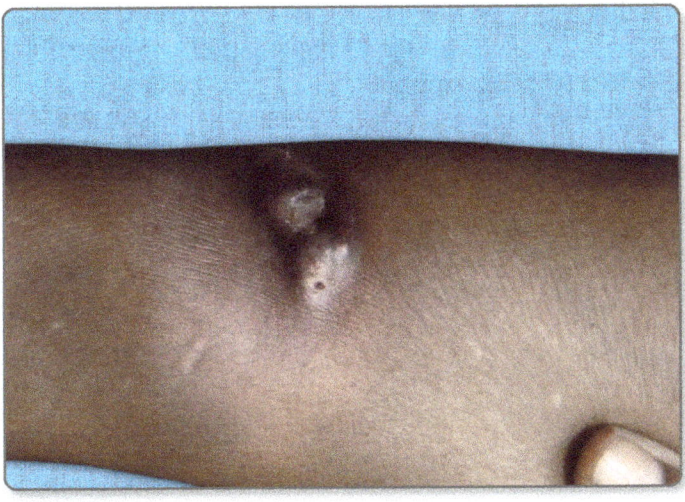

Q. What is the (i) diagnosis and (ii) management?

Answers

i. Erythema induratum of Bazin (if polymerase chain reaction (PCR) from tissue biopsy shows evidence of *Mycobacterium tuberculosis*) or nodular vasculitis (if PCR of *Mycobacterium tuberculosis negative*)

ii. Management:
- Referral to experienced dermatologist
- Management depends on histopathology and PCR report.

Case 51

A 37-year-old lady had frontal alopecia in temporal area with receding hair margin and also severe acne and scar on face for last 6 years. She had also polycystic ovarian disease (PCOD) for last 10 years.

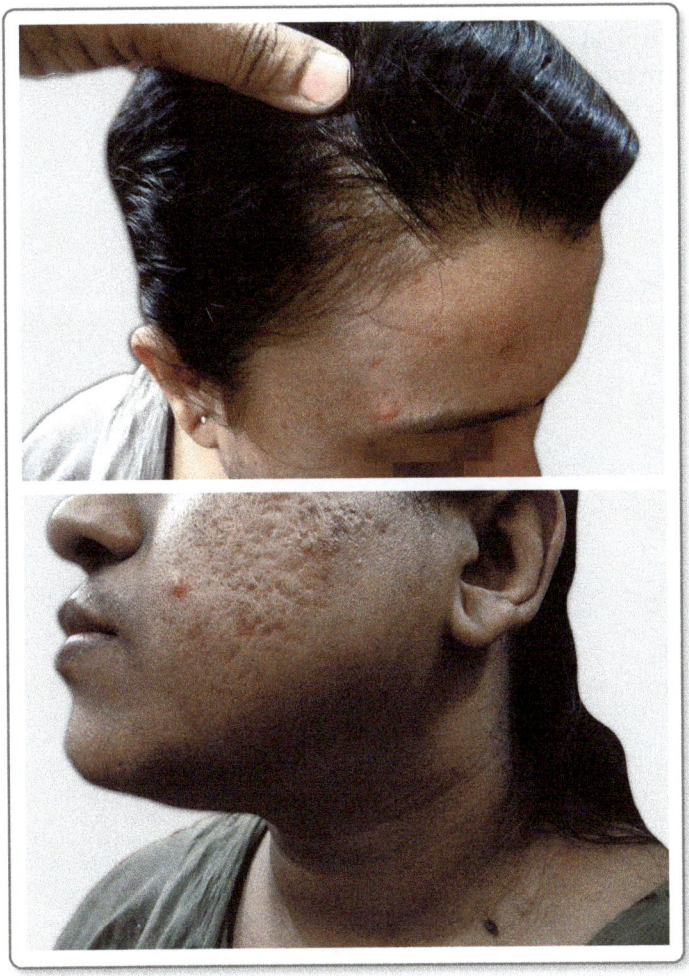

Q. What is the (i) diagnosis and (ii) management?

Answers

i. Male pattern hair loss (Hamilton–Norwood type) and adult acne due to PCOD.
ii. Management:
   - Management of PCOD by gynecologist/endocrinologist
   - Minoxidil 2% lotion 1 mL twice daily on scalp for 6 months
   - Oral doxycycline 100 mg OD or minocycline 100 mg OD or lymecycline 408 mg for 2–3 months
   - Topical benzoyl peroxide, clindamycin, and tretinoin/adaferin on face
   - Acne scar management

Case 52

A 35-year-old lady had extensive hyperpigmented, lichenoid eruptions on limbs for last 5 years. On examination, there were linear arrangement of pigmented papules (white arrows) within the lesion.

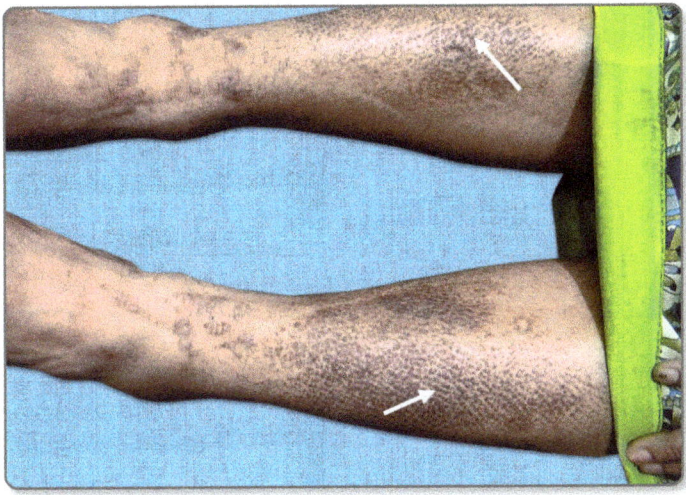

Q. What is the (i) diagnosis and (ii) management?

Answers

i. Lichen amyloid
ii. Management:
   - Avoidance of "bath-scrubbers" on skin
   - Topical potent steroid with or without salicylic acid

Case 53

A 32-year-old male had recurrent boils on different parts of skin for last 3 months. He has no history of diabetes mellitus or any immunosuppressing diseases or drug exposure.

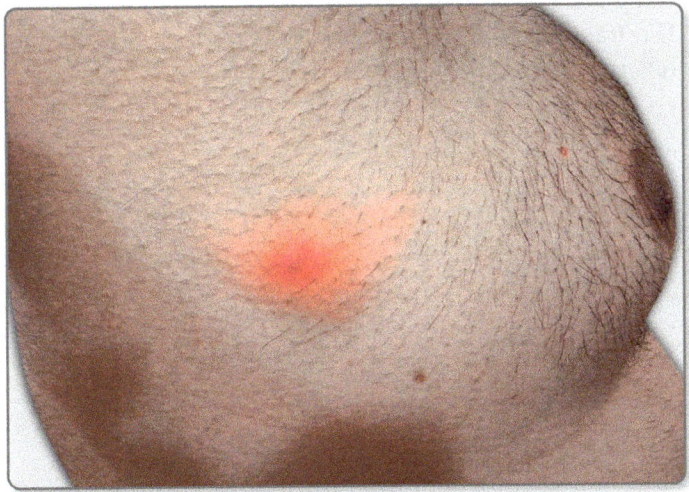

Q. What is the (i) diagnosis and (ii) management?

Answers

i. Recurrent furunculosis
ii. Management:
   - Oral linezolid 600 mg twice daily for 7 days
   - Topical retapamulin twice daily for 7 days
   - Topical mupirocin cream once daily on carrier sites (anterior nares, external auditory meatus, axillae, umbilicus, groin, and inner-buttock cleft) for 7 days/every month for 3 months
   - If refractory, oral rifampicin 450–600 mg orally with amoxicillin 500 mg thrice daily for 10–14 days.

Case 54

A 68-year-old lady had been suffering from recurrent oral ulcer for last 1 year followed by generalized flaccid blister with erosions for last 4 months. On examination, Nikolsky's sign (lateral pressure on skin causes epidermal detachment) was positive (black arrow).

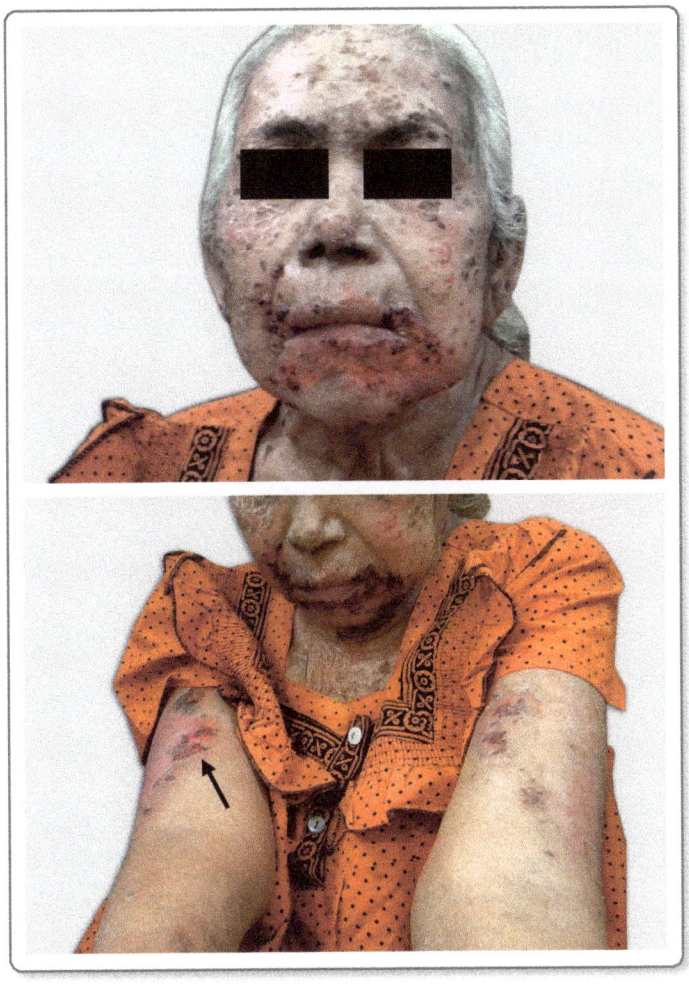

Q. What is the (i) diagnosis and (ii) management?

Answers

i. Pemphigus vulgaris
ii. Management:
   - Referral to expert dermatologist
   - Hospitalization
   - Skin biopsy to confirm the diagnosis
   - High dose of systemic corticosteroids with adjuvants (azathioprine or mycophenolate mofetil) by strict monitoring, or
   - Dexamethasone-cyclophosphamide (DCP) pulse therapy in center where the facility is available.

Case 55

A 32-year-old lady had recurrent painful acneiform eruption on her nape of the neck for last 6 months.

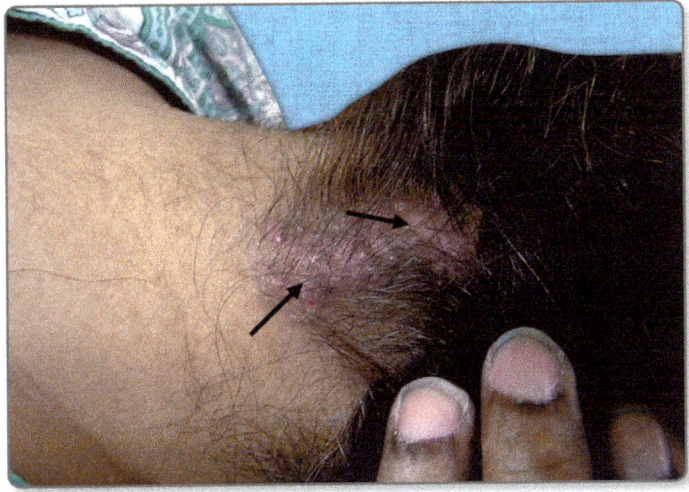

Q. What is the (i) diagnosis and (ii) management?

Answers

i. Acne keloidalis nuchae
ii. Management:
   - Oral doxycycline 100 mg or oral minocycline 100 mg daily or lymecycline 408 mg for 2–3 months
   - Topical benzoyl peroxide or clindamycin gel

Case 56

A lady had asymptomatic pigmented macules and patches for last 2 years on neck and upper trunk. Oral mucosa and nails were not affected.

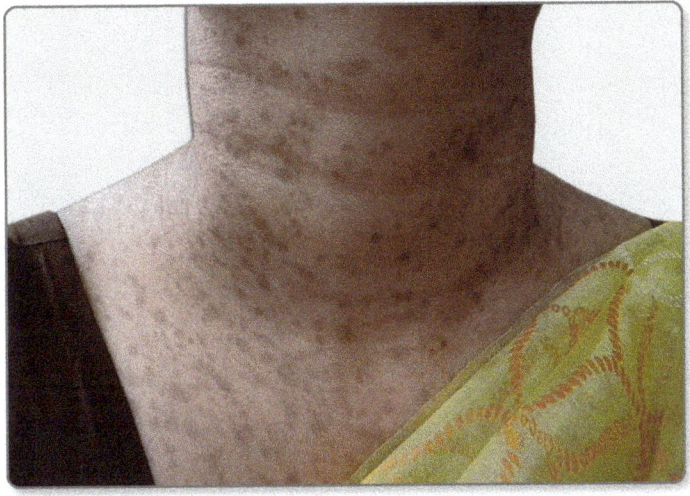

Q. What is the (i) diagnosis and (ii) management?

Answers

i. Lichen planus pigmentosus
ii. Management:
   - Broad-spectrum sunscreen
   - Topical mid-potent corticosteroid

Case 57

A 19-year-old girl had excessive sweating on hands and feet for last 5 years. She felt difficulty in writing and computer typing.

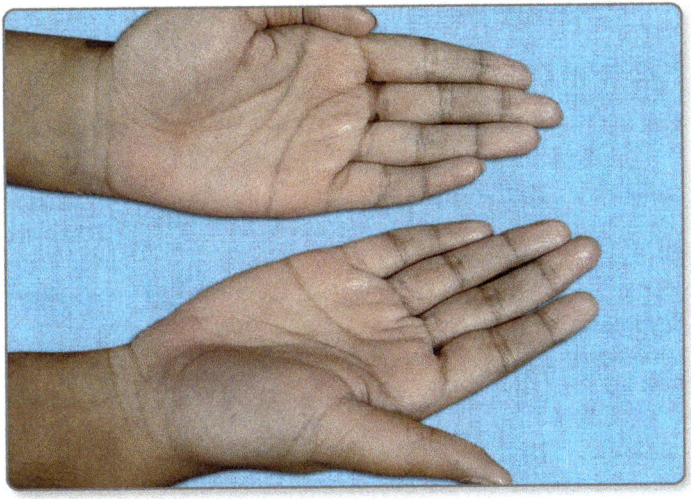

Q. What is the (i) diagnosis and (ii) management?

Answers

i. Palmoplantar hyperhidrosis
ii. Management:
    - Stress control
    - Topical aluminum chloride hexahydrate 20% in absolute alcohol to apply once at night
    - Tap water iontophoresis

Case 58

A 51-year-old male asymptomatic, persistent, glistening moist shiny reddish patches on glans and inner prepuce (black arrows) for last 2 years.

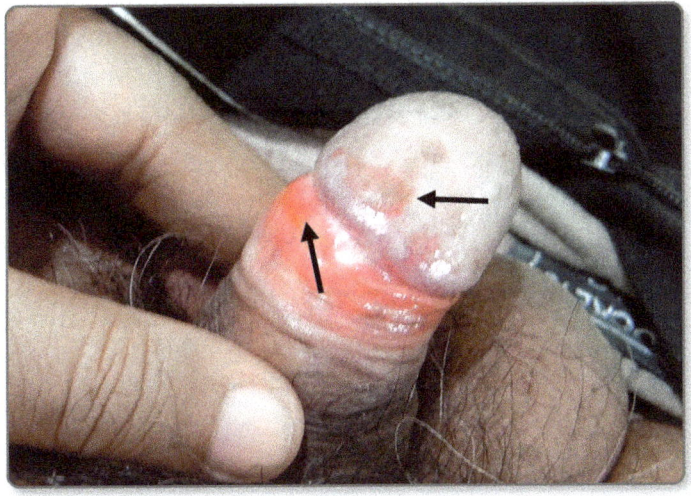

Q. What is the (i) diagnosis and (ii) management?

Answers

i. Zoon's (plasma cell) balanitis
ii. Management:
   - To improve washing habits and micturition practices
   - Intermittent application of mild to potent topical corticosteroids with or without antibacterials and antifungals
   - Topical tacrolimus
   - In refractory cases, surgical circumcision

Case 59

A 61-year-old male had recurrent painful pustular lesions on upper lip and beard for last 1 year. On examination, perifollicular inflammation was seen.

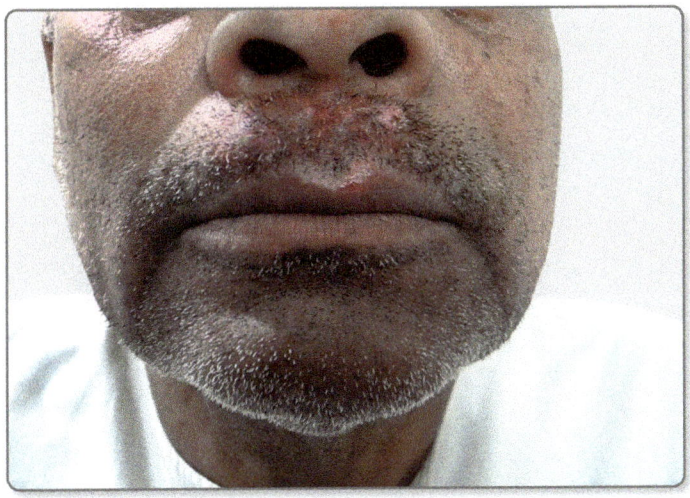

Q. What is the (i) diagnosis and (ii) management?

Answers

i. Sycosis barbae
ii. Management:
   - Warm saline compress
   - Avoid saloon shaving
   - Local antibiotic (ozenoxacin, mupirocin, or clindamycin)
   - Systemic antibiotic

Case 60

A 28-year-old male had recurrent painful vesicular lesions followed by superficial erosions (black arrows) on glans for last 2 years. He had extramarital partner.

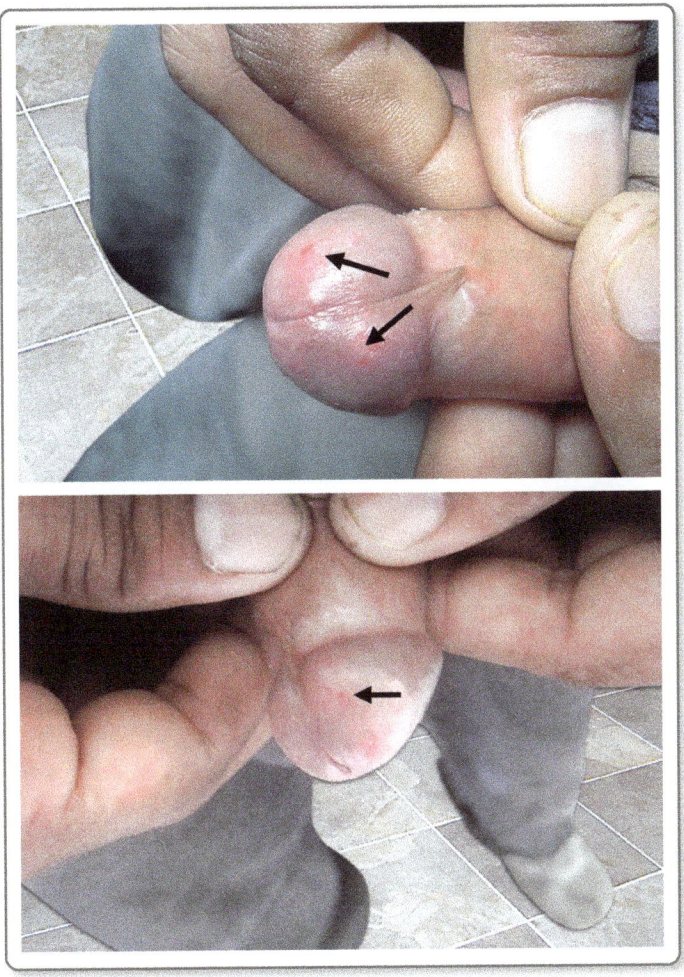

Q. What is the (i) diagnosis and (ii) management?

Answers

i. Recurrent herpes genitalis
ii. Management:
   - To screen for other sexually transmitted diseases (STDs), especially HIV
   - Suppressive treatment (if recurrence 6 incidents/year):
     - Oral valacyclovir 500 mg daily or 1,000 mg daily
     - Or oral acyclovir 400 mg twice daily
     - Or oral famciclovir 250 mg twice daily
   - Treatment duration: Up to 1 year

Case 61

A 61-year-old male had tingling and numbness on anterolateral aspect of left thigh (on marked area) for last 6 months. On examination, neither any skin patch nor any nerve thickening was detected.

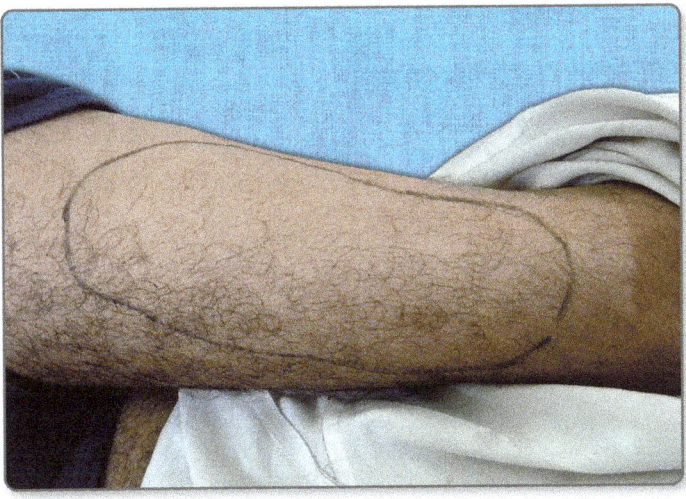

Q. What is the (i) diagnosis and (ii) management?

Answers

i. Meralgia paresthetica (Bernhardt's syndrome)
ii. Management:
    ➢ Referral to orthopedic surgeon/neurologist

Case 62

A 27-year-old male had asymptomatic progressively increasing generalized hypopigmented patches mostly on nonexposed skin for last 4 years.

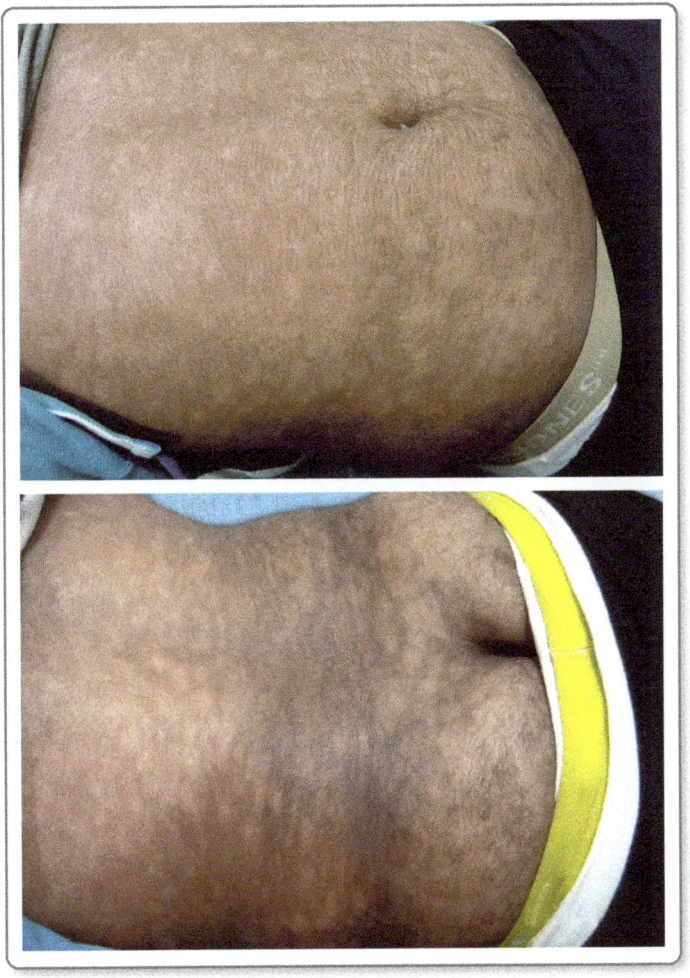

Q. What is the (i) diagnosis and (ii) management?

Answers

i. Mycosis fungoides (cutaneous T-cell lymphoma)
ii. Management:
   - Referral to experienced dermatologist
   - To confirm diagnosis by histopathology and immunohistopathology
   - Staging of the disease
   - Psoralen plus ultraviolet A (PUVA) therapy or topical bexarotene or electron beam
   - Systemic chemotherapy

Case 63

A 27-year-old male had multiple pruritic, erythematous papulovesicles (black arrows) on different parts of trunk and limbs for last 1 week. On examination, the lesions had central puncta with surrounding areola (white arrow).

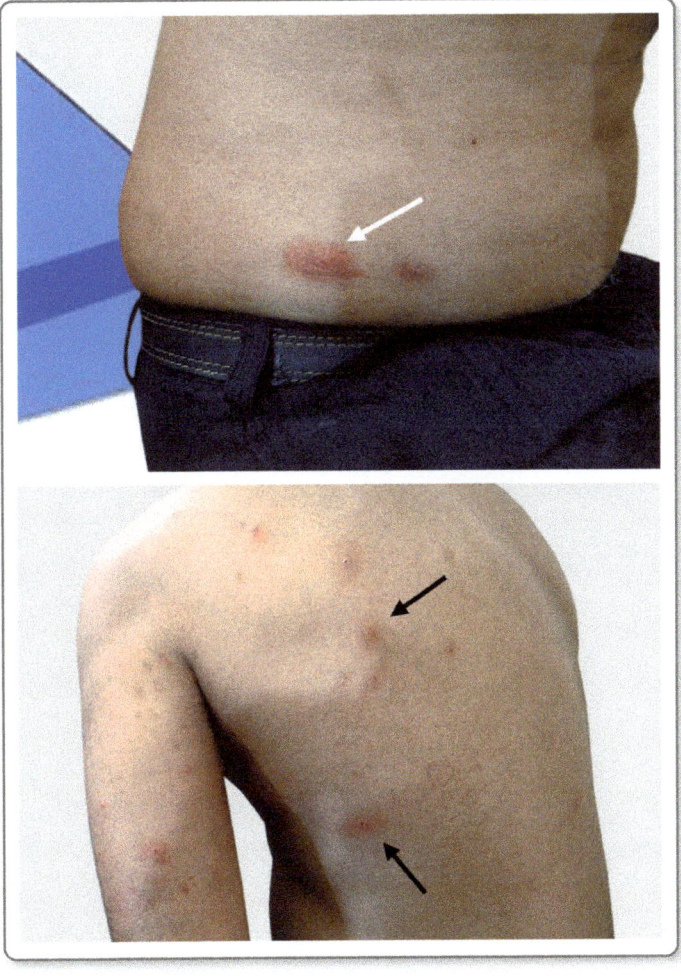

Q. What is the (i) diagnosis and (ii) management?

Answers

i. Insect allergy
ii. Management:
    - To avoid insect exposure
    - Topical mid-potent steroid with or without antibacterials
    - Oral antihistamines

Case 64

A 56-year-old lady had pruritic annular lesion on face for last 3 months. On examination, the active border (black arrow) of the lesions showed papulovesicles and scales.

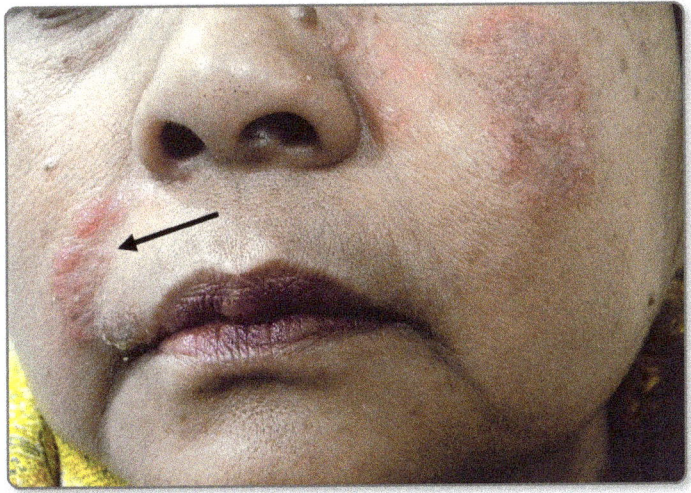

Q. What is the (i) diagnosis and (ii) management?

Answers

i. Tinea faciei
ii. Management:
   - Oral itraconazole 200 mg OD for 14 days:
     - Or oral terbinafine 250 mg OD for 14 days
     - Or oral fluconazole 150 mg once/week for 4 weeks
   - Topical luliconazole, oxiconazole, amorolfine, or clotrimazole daily for 4 weeks
   - Maintenance of hygiene (changing/washing/ironing of inner garments, not sharing of clothes, separate washing of clothes, etc.)

Case 65

A 17-year-old male had generalized asymptomatic nodules (black arrow), freckles (white arrows), and Café au lait macules (blue arrow) on different parts of trunk and limbs.

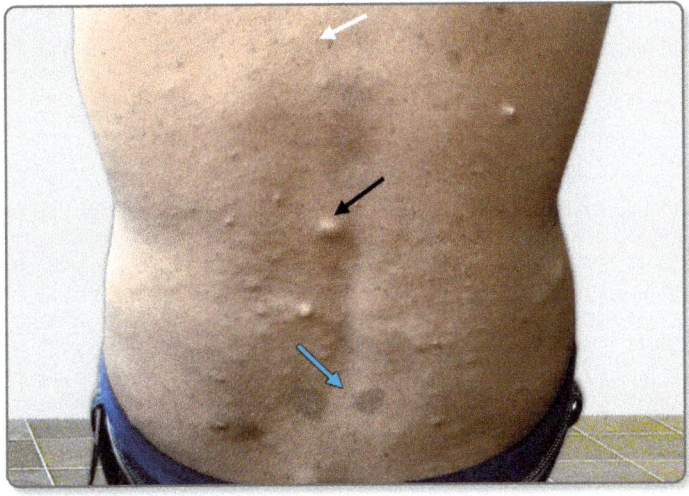

Q. What is the (i) diagnosis and (ii) management?

Answers

i. Neurofibromatosis
ii. Management:
   - Counseling
   - Referral to neurologist to exclude intracerebral involvement (CT scan, MRI, etc.).

Case 66

A 32-year-old male had severe pruritus on scrotum for last 2 years. On examination, the scrotal skin showed lichenification.

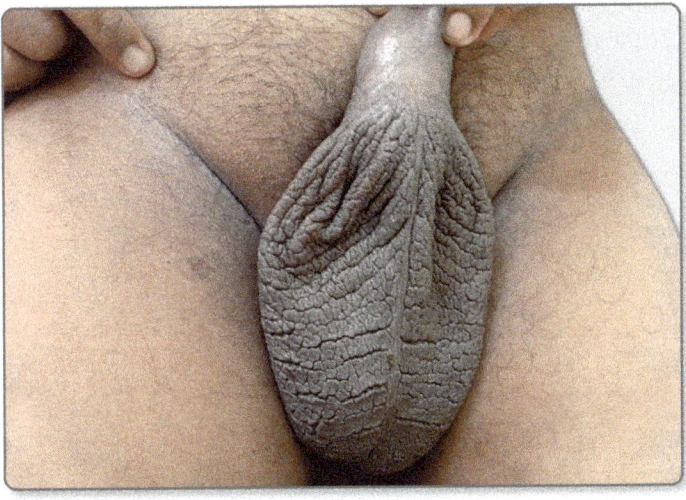

Q. What is the (i) diagnosis and (ii) management?

Answers

i. Scrotal dermatitis
ii. Management:
    - To avoid synthetic underwears, strong washing agents for underclothes
    - Stress control
    - Topical emollients (without fragrances, lanolin, and paraben)
    - Topical low potent steroids or tacrolimus or pimecrolimus
    - Oral antihistamines

Case 67

A 25-year-old male had asymptomatic hypopigmented lesions on trunk and limbs for last 3 years mostly aggravating during summer and rainy season. On examination, satellite lesions and perifollicular lesions were seen.

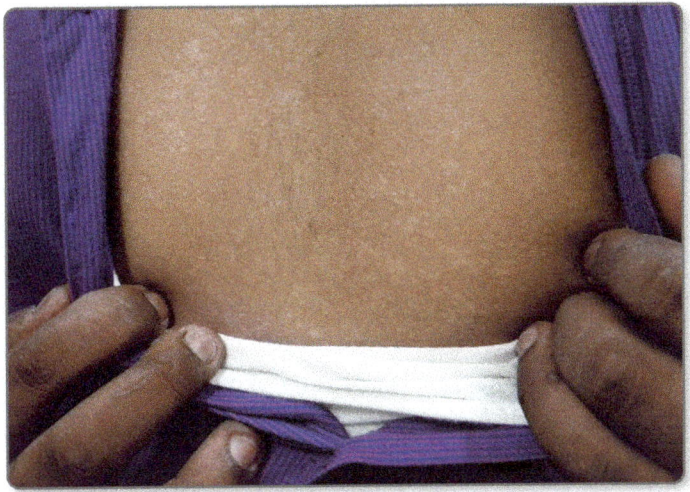

Q. What is the (i) diagnosis and (ii) management?

Answers

i. Pityriasis versicolor
ii. Management:
   - Topical 2% ketoconazole shampoo to apply for 5 minutes before bath for 3 consecutive days.
   - *Oral antifungals*: Ketoconazole 200 mg daily for 7 days or itraconazole 100–200 mg twice daily for 7 days or fluconazole 400 mg stat.

Case 68

A 3-year-old child had recurrent pruritic popular and papulovesicular lesions mostly on exposed skin (especially both legs and forearms) for last 2 years. On examination, many lesions were excoriated.

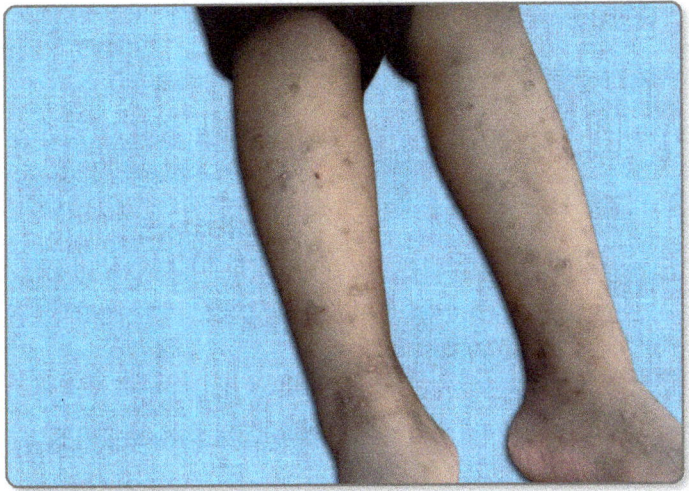

Q. What is the (i) diagnosis and (ii) management?

Answers

i. Papular urticaria
ii. Management:
   - To avoid insects (especially mosquito) exposure
   - To use full sleeves
   - Topical calamine lotion
   - Oral antihistamines
   - Short course of antibiotics, if secondary infection

Case 69

A 34-year-old male had recurrent painful boils like swelling on axillae and groins for last 4 years.

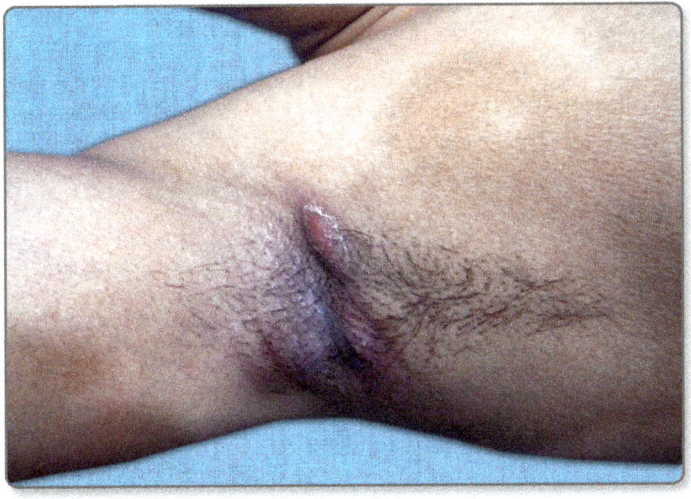

Q. What is the (i) diagnosis and (ii) management?

Answers

i. Hidradenitis suppurativa
ii. Management:
   - Weight reduction, loose clothes, avoiding friction, and moisture accumulation
   - Topical clindamycin for 3 months
   - Systemic tetracycline 250–500 mg four times daily until lesions resolved
     - Or systemic erythromycin 250–500 mg four times daily until lesions resolved
     - Or oral minocycline 100 mg twice daily until lesions resolved
   - Surgery in certain cases

Case 70

A 6-month-old child had depigmented lesion on abdomen since birth. On examination, the lesion sharply demarcated (black arrow) at midline and outer border was bizarre or map-like (blue arrow). On diascopy, the lesional border became more distinct.

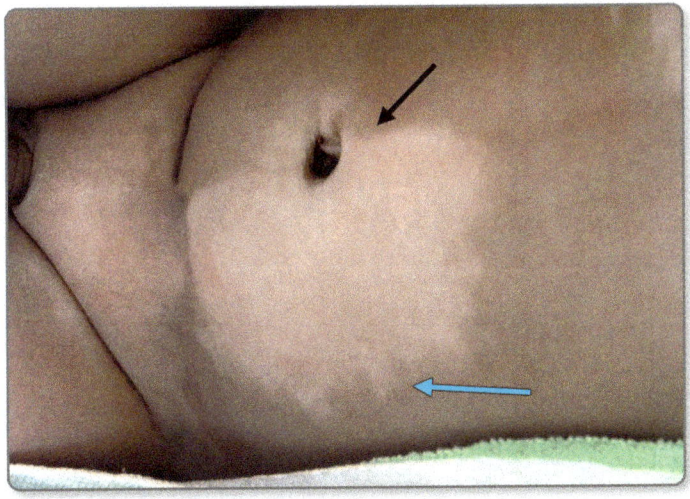

Q. What is the (i) diagnosis and (ii) management?

Answers

i. Nevus depigmentosus
ii. Management:
   - Counseling
   - Watch by mapping
   - Covermark

Case 71

A 35-year-old male had chronic pruritic lichenified eczematous lesions on palm of the both hands for last 1 year. He had history of contact with cement as construction supervisor.

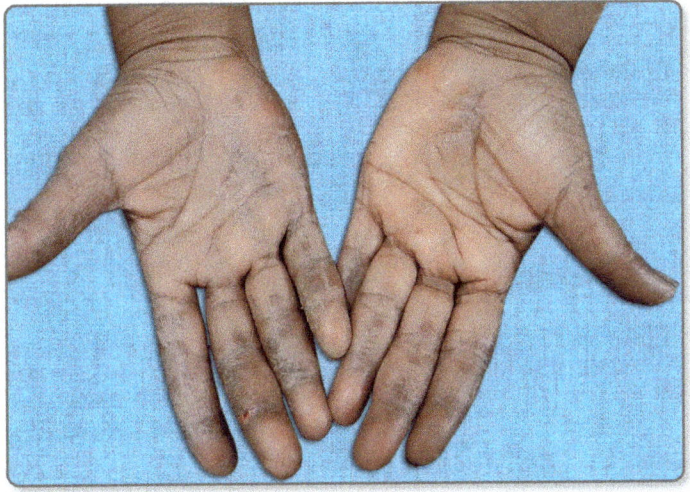

Q. What is the (i) diagnosis and (ii) management?

Answers

i. Contact dermatitis (probably from cement)
ii. Management:
   - Confirmation of cause of contact dermatitis by allergic patch test
   - To use glove/barrier cream while in contact with cement
   - Use mild hand wash
   - To use emollient liberally
   - Potent to super potent topical corticosteroid twice daily followed by mid-potent steroid or tacrolimus ointment
   - Oral antihistaminic

Case 72

A 61-year-old male had asymptomatic depigmented patches on lips, hands, and feet for last 5 years, which were not progressive.

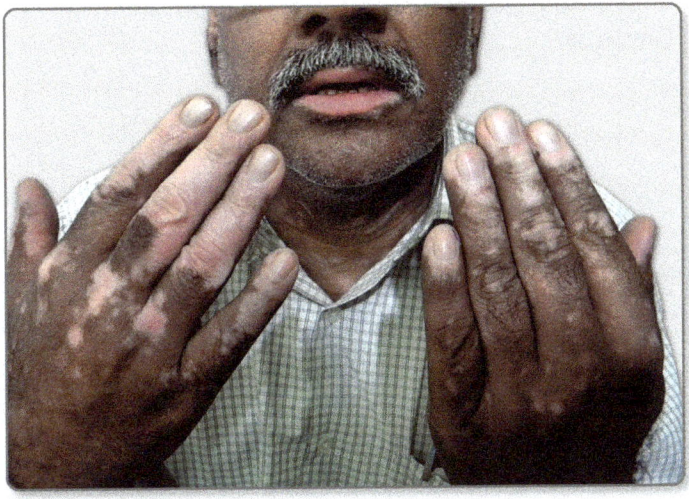

Q. What is the (i) diagnosis and (ii) management?

Answers

i. Vitiligo (lip-tip variety)
ii. Management:
   - Counseling
   - Ultraviolet B (UVB) narrow band or PUVA therapy or excimer light/laser under experienced dermatologist
     - Or PUVAsol (oral psoralen + sun exposure)
   - Covermark

Case 73

An 18-year-old male had asymptomatic yellowish nodules (black arrow) on elbows and knees for last 2 months. He had family history of dyslipidemia.

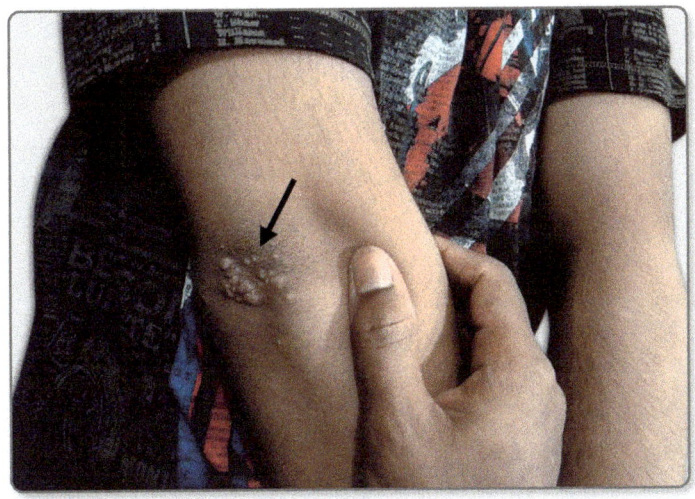

Q. What is the (i) diagnosis and (ii) management?

Answers

i. Eruptive xanthoma
ii. Management:
   - Screening for dyslipidemia
   - Management of dyslipidemia by physician

Case 74

A 35-year-old lady had multiple asymptomatic umbilicated papules (black arrows) on face for last 3 months. She had history of frequent exposure to beauty parlor for different procedures.

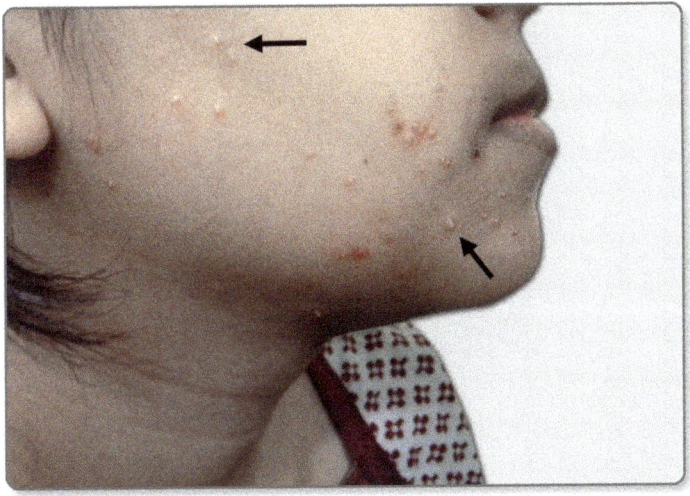

Q. What is the (i) diagnosis and (ii) management?

Answers

i. Molluscum contagiosum
ii. Management:
   - Extraction and iodine cautery or light electrofulguration

Case 75

A 67-year-old male had whitish plaque on glans and prepuce, which had been gradually tightened during 3 years producing acquired phimosis. The patient had also partly narrowing of his urine stream.

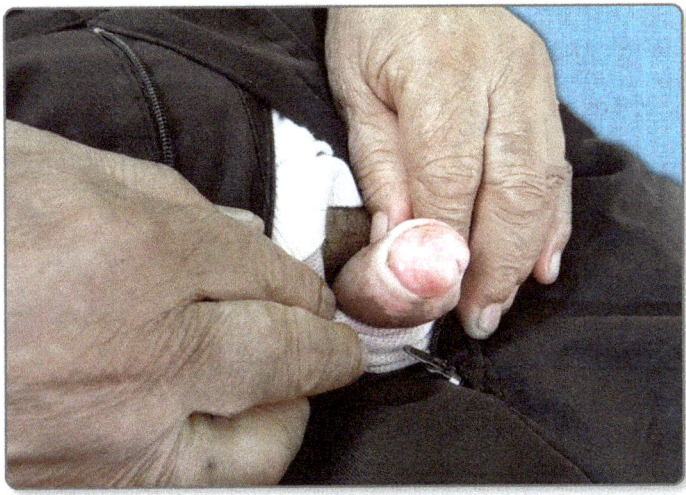

Q. What is the (i) diagnosis and (ii) management?

Answers

i. Lichen sclerosus et atrophicus (LSA) or balanitis xerotica obliterans (BXO).
ii. Management:
   - Circumcision and biopsy from the glans by urosurgeon
   - Urethral dilatation, if needed

Case 76

A 39-year-old male had nail dystrophy (white arrows), namely subungual hyperkeratosis, thickening and discoloration of nail plate, on multiple fingers and toes for last 3 years. He had history of diabetes.

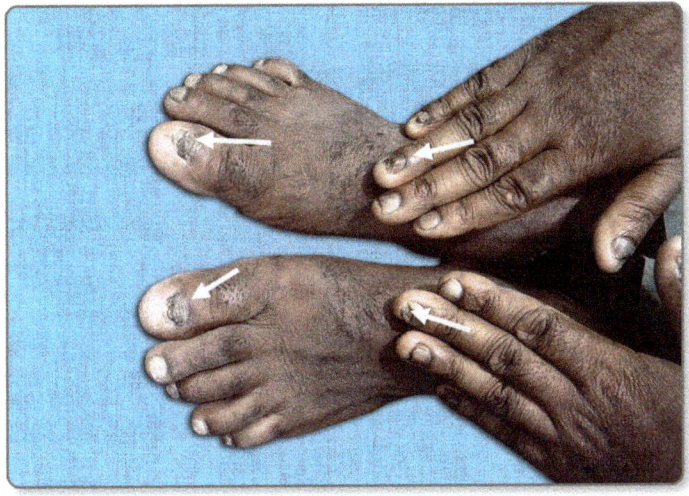

Q. What is the (i) diagnosis and (ii) management?

Answers

i. Tinea unguium or onychomycosis
ii. Management:
   - Oral terbinafine 250 mg daily for 6 weeks
     - Or oral itraconazole 200 mg twice daily for 7 days to repeat the pulse for 2 (for fingers) to 3 months (for toes)
     - Or oral fluconazole 150 mg once in a week for 3–6 months
   - Topical amorolfine lacquer once in a week for 3 months

Case 77

A 64-year-old lady suddenly developed frontal baldness for last 6 months. On investigations, she had shown high dehydroepiandrosterone sulfate (DHEAS) level and adrenal tumor by ultrasonography.

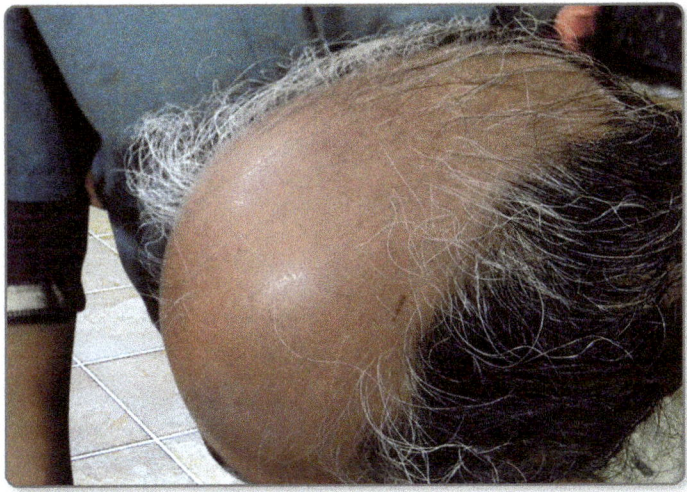

Q. What is the (i) diagnosis and (ii) management?

Answers

i. Androgenetic alopecia due to adrenal tumor
ii. Management:
   - Referral to endocrinologist
   - Topical minoxidil 2% lotion 1 mL twice daily

Case 78

A 65-year-old male had sudden development of asymptomatic reddish macules and patches on trunk and limbs for last 1 week. On investigations, his platelet count was 45,000/μL.

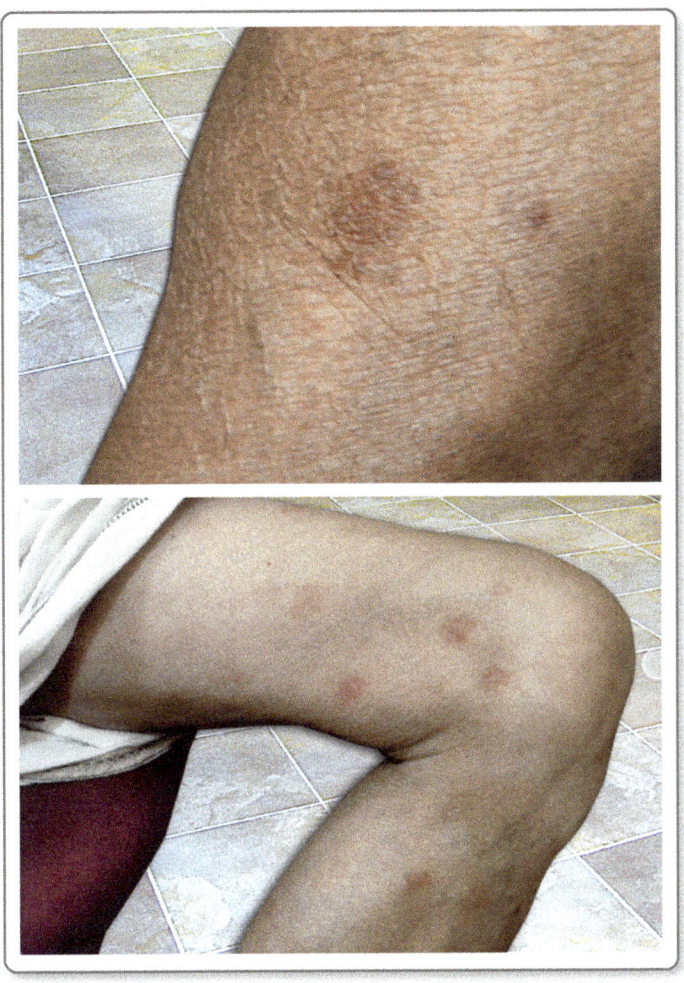

Q. What is the (i) diagnosis and (ii) management?

Answers

i. Thrombocytopenic purpura
ii. Management:
   - Referral to hematologist

Case 79

A 29-year-old male had mild scaly plaques on scrotum and glans for last 6 months. He had also scaly plaques on elbows, knees, and different parts of trunk and nail pitting.

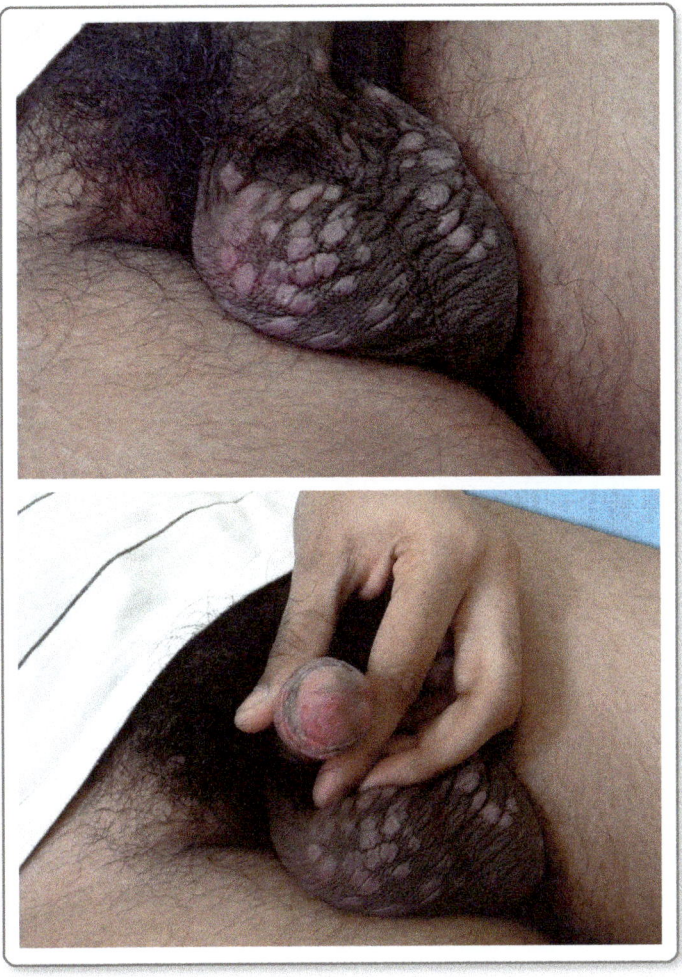

Q. What is the (i) diagnosis and (ii) management?

Answers

i. Psoriasis on scrotum and glans
ii. Management:
    - Topical low potent corticosteroid once daily
    - Or topical tacrolimus 0.1% or pimecrolimus 1% twice daily.

Case 80

A 23-year-old male had extensive scaly xerotic pruritic lesion almost all over the body for last 3 months. He had history of chronic pruritic flexural dermatitis along with bronchial asthma since childhood. After taking oral steroids for 6 months sudden withdrawal had converted the limited lesions into extensive one.

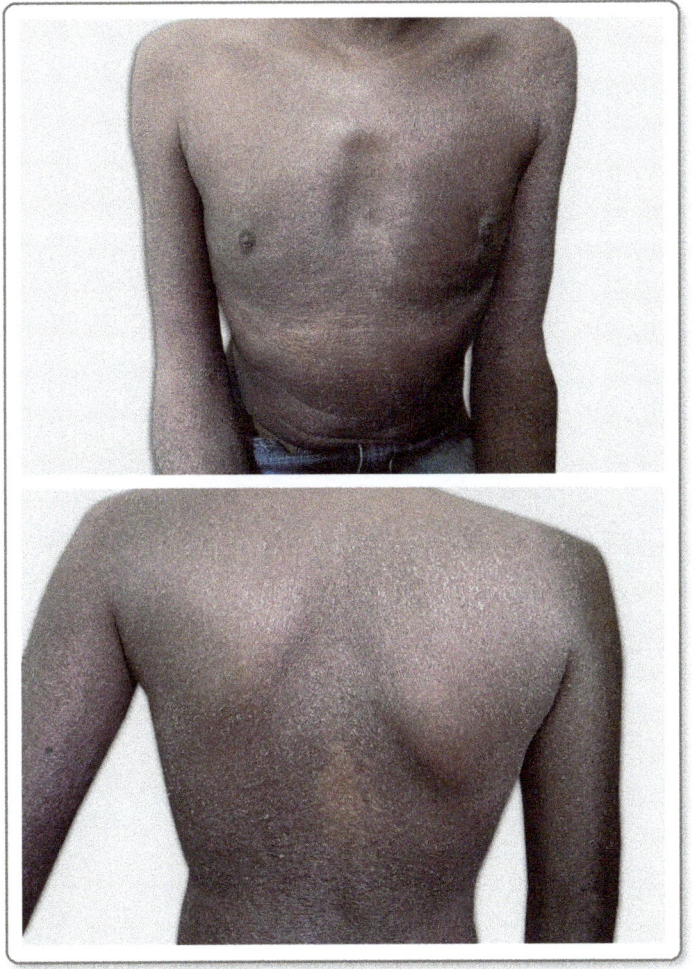

Q. What is the (i) diagnosis and (ii) management?

Answers

i. Exfoliative dermatitis or erythroderma due to atopic dermatitis.
ii. Management:
   - Management of erythroderma by admission, fluid-electrolyte and temperature balance, nutrition care, and emollient application
   - Treatment of secondary infection
   - *Specific treatment of atopic dermatitis*: Oral steroids or oral cyclosporine, etc., under expert dermatologist

Case 81

A 21-year-old female had asymptomatic small scaly (lid-like scale) eruption (blue arrow) followed by hypopigmented patches (black arrow) for last 1 year.

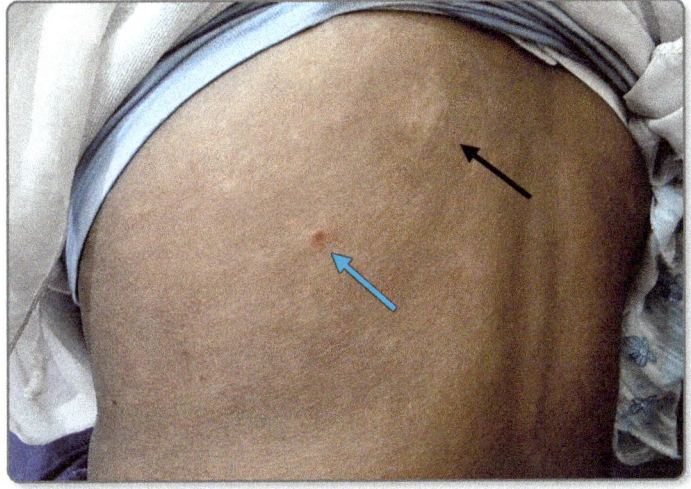

Q. What is the (i) diagnosis and (ii) management?

Answers

i. Pityriasis lichenoides chronica
ii. Management:
   - Referral to dermatologist
   - Narrow band UVB (NB-UVB), PUVA, or PUVAsol therapy
   - Topical steroid

Case 82

A 21-year-old young man had inflammatory papules, pustules, and comedones like eruption for last 3 years.

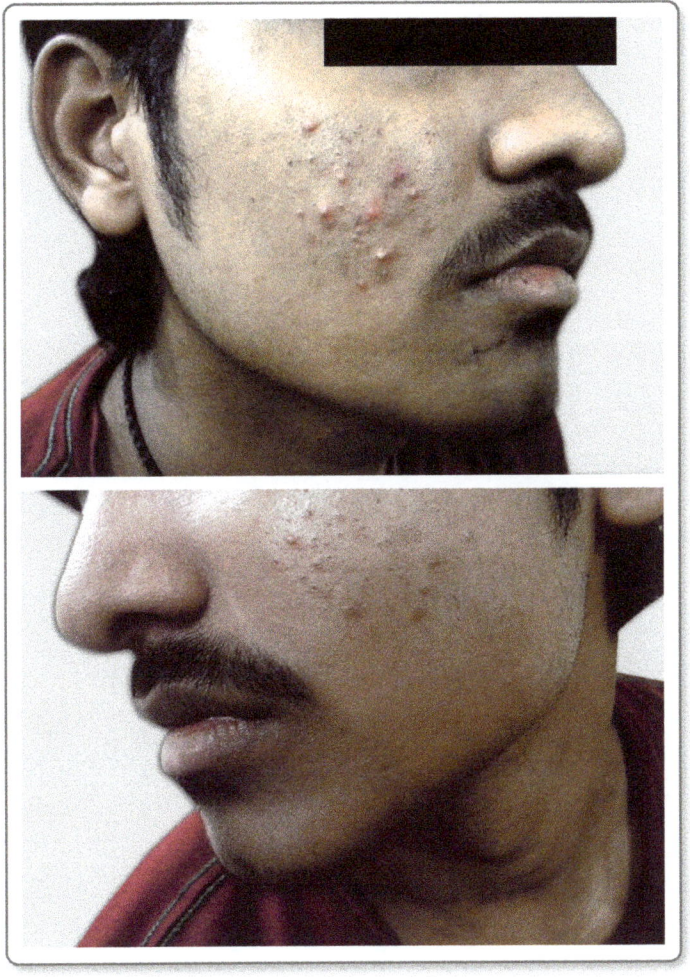

Q. What is the (i) diagnosis and (ii) management?

Answers

i. Acne vulgaris
ii. Management:
   - Oral tetracycline 500 mg TID or doxycycline 100 mg daily or minocycline 100 or lymecycline 408 mg daily up to 3 months
   - Topical clindamycin, benzoyl peroxide 2.5% gel or wash, and tretinoin or adapalene

Case 83

A 34-year-old female had localized scarring alopecia for last 3 years, which was gradually increasing in size. On examination, the lesion showed prominent follicular keratosis and atrophy.

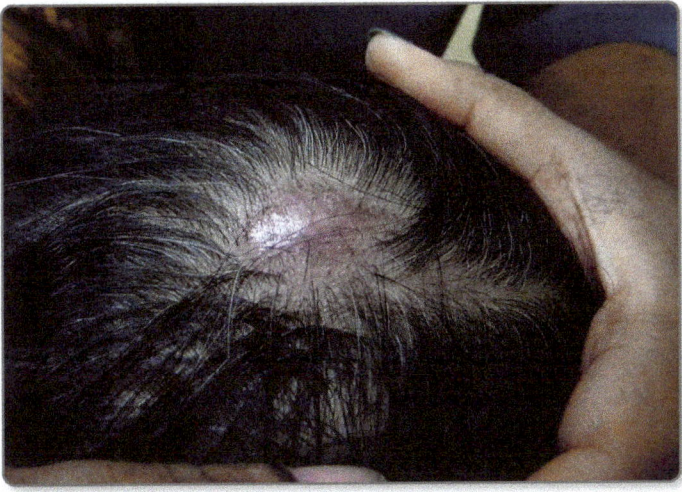

Q. What is the (i) diagnosis and (ii) management?

Answers

i. Cicatricial alopecia due to discoid lupus erythematosus (DLE).
ii. Management:
   - Avoidance of daylight
   - Use of sunscreen/cap/umbrella
   - Screening for systemic lupus erythematosus (SLE)
   - Oral hydroxychloroquine 200–400 mg daily under experienced dermatologist with pre- and per-therapy eye screening.

Case 84

A 31-year-old male had asymptomatic pigmented patches on both axillae for last 6 months. Neither any perifollicular lesion nor any satellite lesions was observed.

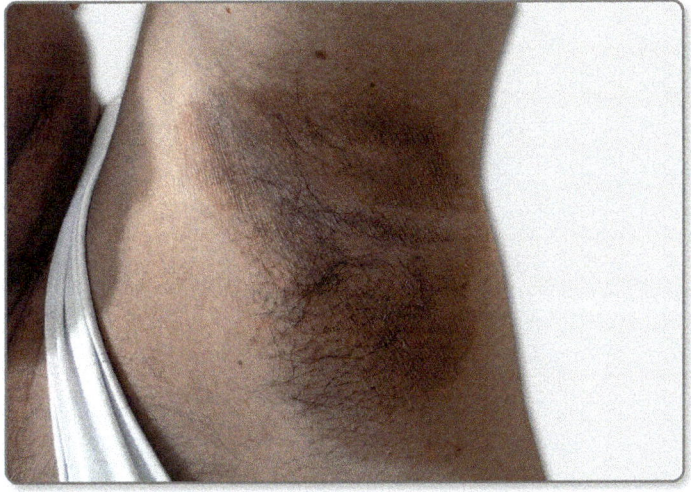

Q. What is the (i) diagnosis and (ii) management?

Answers

i. Erythrasma
ii. Management:
    - Topical benzoyl peroxide 2.5% gel or wash
    - Topical clindamycin or miconazole gel
    - If refractory, oral erythromycin 250 mg four times daily for 7 days

Case 85

A 58-year-old lady had chronic eczematous lesions on the tips of her fingers for last 2 years. She had regular habit of contact with different flowers during worship and also different vegetables during cooking.

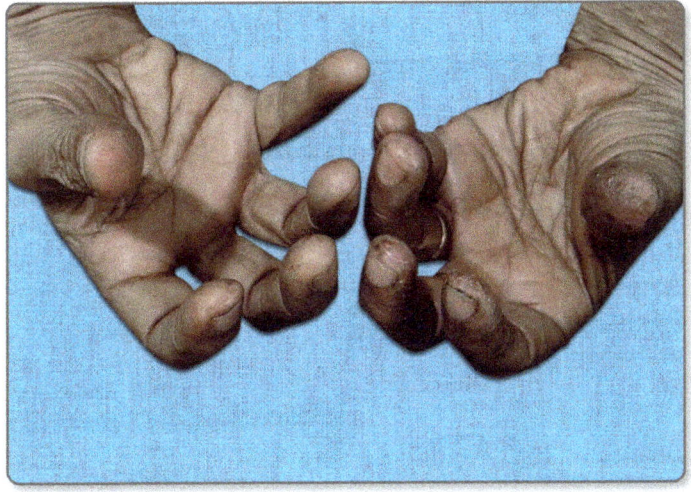

Q. What is the (i) diagnosis and (ii) management?

Answers

i. Contact dermatitis from flowers/vegetables
ii. Management:
   - Avoidance of contact allergens
   - Topical steroids

Case 86

A 41-year-old lady had asymptomatic pigmented patches (white arrows) on neck, upper chest, and back for last 6 months. She was a frequent user of fragrances by spray on neck and upper trunk.

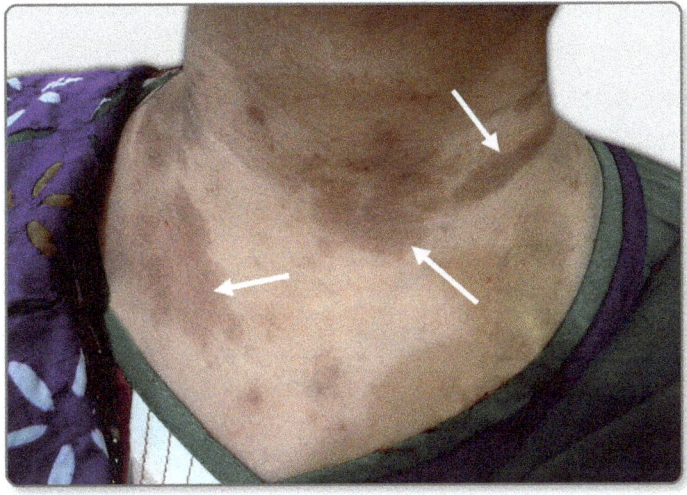

Q. What is the (i) diagnosis and (ii) management?

Answers

i. Pigmented contact dermatitis from fragrances.
ii. Management:
   - Avoidance of fragrances
   - Topical steroids
   - Broad-spectrum sunscreen
   - Patch testing

Case 87

A 65-year-old male had sudden loss of hair for last 2 months producing circumscribed area of alopecia, which did not show any scarring.

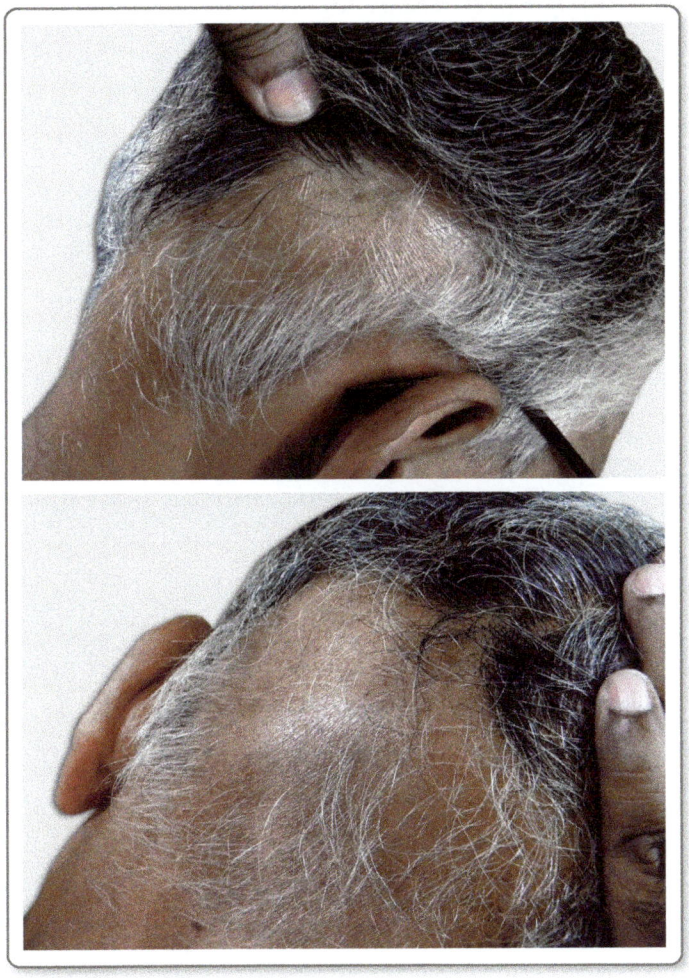

Q. What is the (i) diagnosis and (ii) management?

Answers

i. Alopecia areata
ii. Management:
   - Topical super potent corticosteroid or intralesional triamcinolone by expert dermatologist.
   - If refractory, contact immunotherapy by diphenylcyclopropenone (DPCP) by expert dermatologists.

Case 88

A 38-year-old female had painful hyperkeratotic lesions (black arrows) on different parts of the feet for last 5 years. On examination, the lesions were more tender on ventral pressure than lateral pressure.

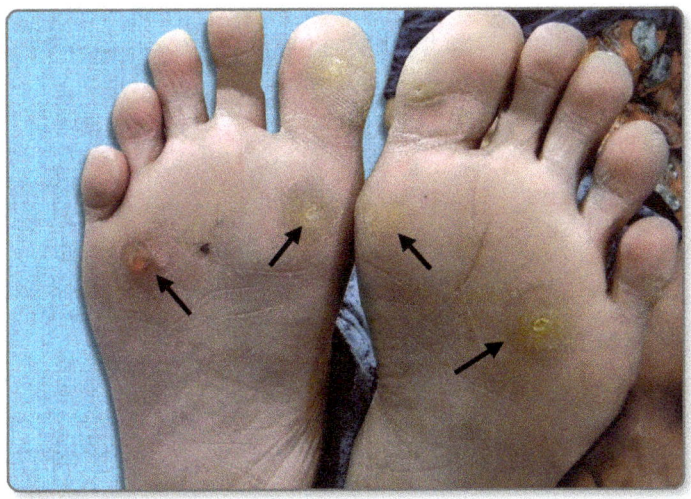

Q. What is the (i) diagnosis and (ii) management?

Answers

i. Plantar corn (callosity)
ii. Management:
    - Proper shoe
    - Salicylic acid 16.5%
    - Lactic acid 16.5%
    - Collodion flexile 25 mL
    - Mft pig
    - Apply at night with applicator only on corns

Case 89

A 46-year-old lady had chronic dry lesions (black arrows) on palms, especially in between fingers for last 3 years. She had history of frequent water and soap wash of hands.

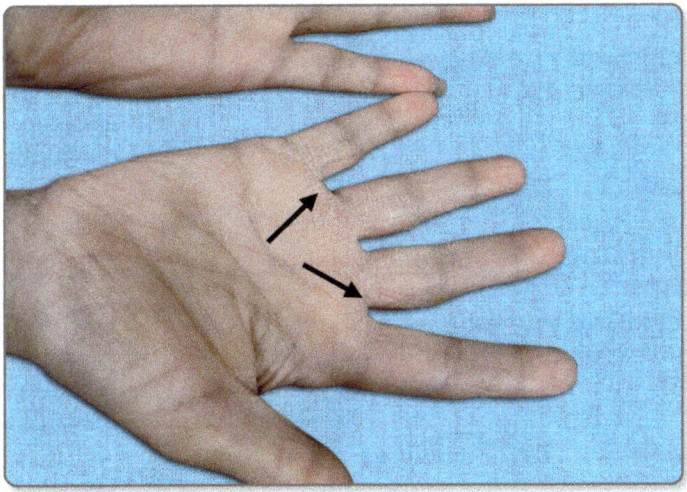

Q. What is the (i) diagnosis and (ii) management?

Answers

i. Irritant contact dermatitis (chronic cumulative)
ii. Management:
   - Restricted soap and water use
   - Liberal use of emollients
   - Topical potent steroids

Case 90

A lady had chronic erosion on tongue for last 5 years, which on examination, showed erythematous raw area with loss of papillae and sharp whitish circinate or serpiginous border.

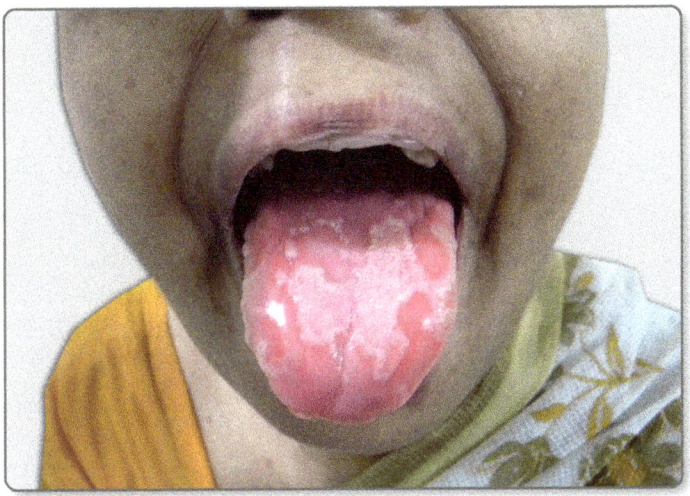

Q. What is the (i) diagnosis and (ii) management?

Answers

i. Geographic tongue
ii. Management:
   - Counseling
   - Topical lignocaine for pain relieve
   - Clotrimazole troche to suck twice daily to control secondary candidiasis

Case 91

A 31-year-old lady had asymptomatic thick yellowish plaques on both eyelids for last 1 year. She had family history of similar lesions.

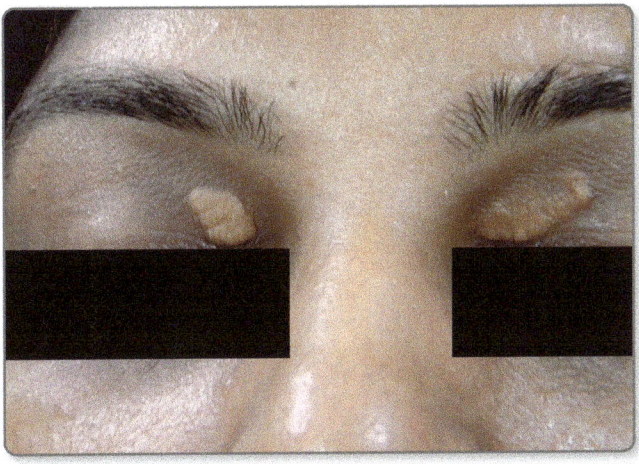

Q. What is the (i) diagnosis and (ii) management?

Answers

i. Xanthelasma palpebrarum
ii. Management:
    - Screening serum lipid profile
    - Counseling
    - Topical trichloroacetic acid (TCA) application by expert dermatologist

Case 92

A 51-year-old female had asymptomatic pigmented patches on both cheeks for last 2 years.

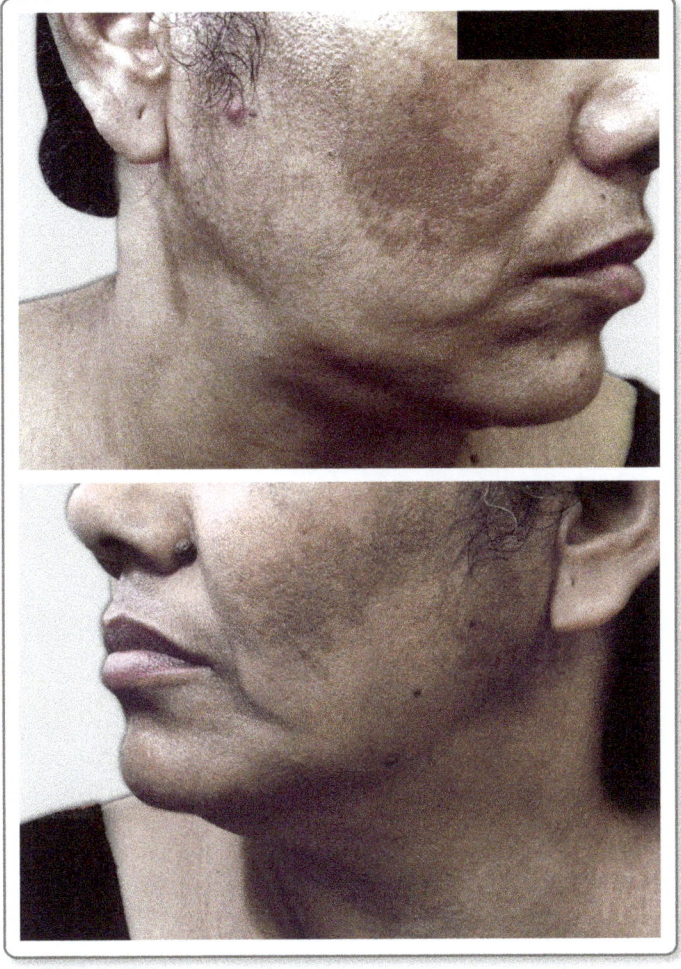

Q. What is the (i) diagnosis and (ii) management?

Answers

i. Melasma
ii. Management:
   - Broad spectrum sunscreen
   - Topical tretinoin 0.025% or topical kojic acid 2% or glycolic acid 6%

Case 93

A 29-year-old lady had papulovesicular eruptions on both forearms, V-area of neck, and back of neck for last 2 weeks at the end of the spring. She had similar eruptions at same sites during the same time for last 2 years.

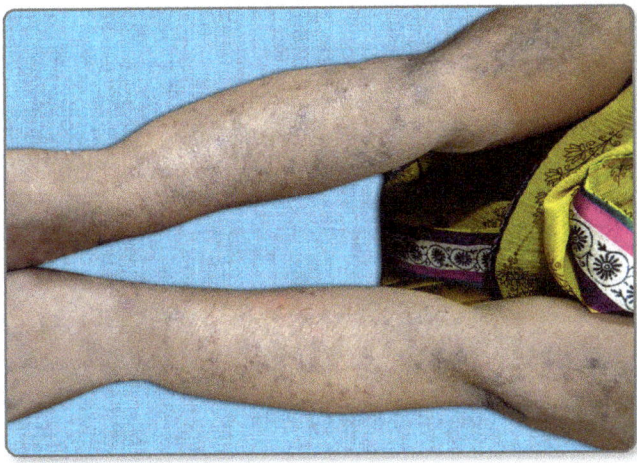

Q. What is the (i) diagnosis and (ii) management?

Answers

i. Polymorphous light eruption
ii. Management:
   - Avoidance of daylight
   - Topical mid-potent steroids/topical tacrolimus
   - Antihistamines
   - Broad-spectrum sunscreen

Case 94

A 51-year-old lady had superficial pustular eruptions often in annular distribution mostly in intertriginous area (axillae, inframammary, and groin) for last 5 years.

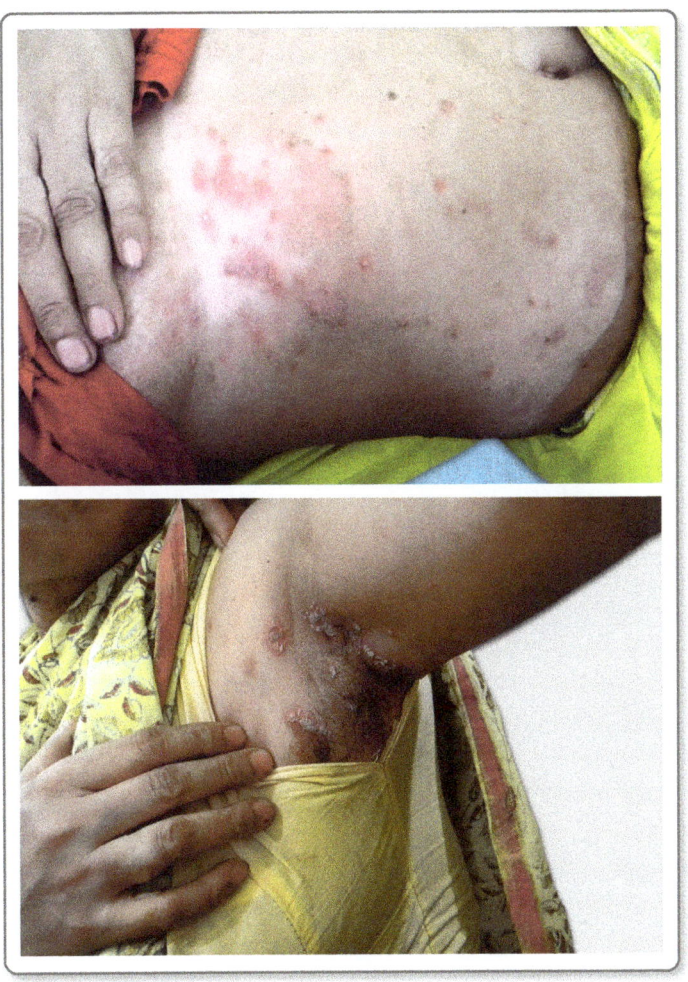

Q. What is the (i) diagnosis and (ii) management?

Answers

i. Subcorneal pustular dermatoses (SCPD)
ii. Management:
   - Referral to competent dermatologist
   - Confirmation by histopathology test
   - Dapsone under dermatologist's supervision by previous glucose-6-phosphate dehydrogenase (G6PD) screening (quantitative)
   - Or oral isotretinoin under expert dermatologists

Case 95

A 31-year-old male had extensive papulosquamous skin eruption involving scalp, eyelids, postauricular region, front of the chest and back (interscapular region), and groin for last 5 years.

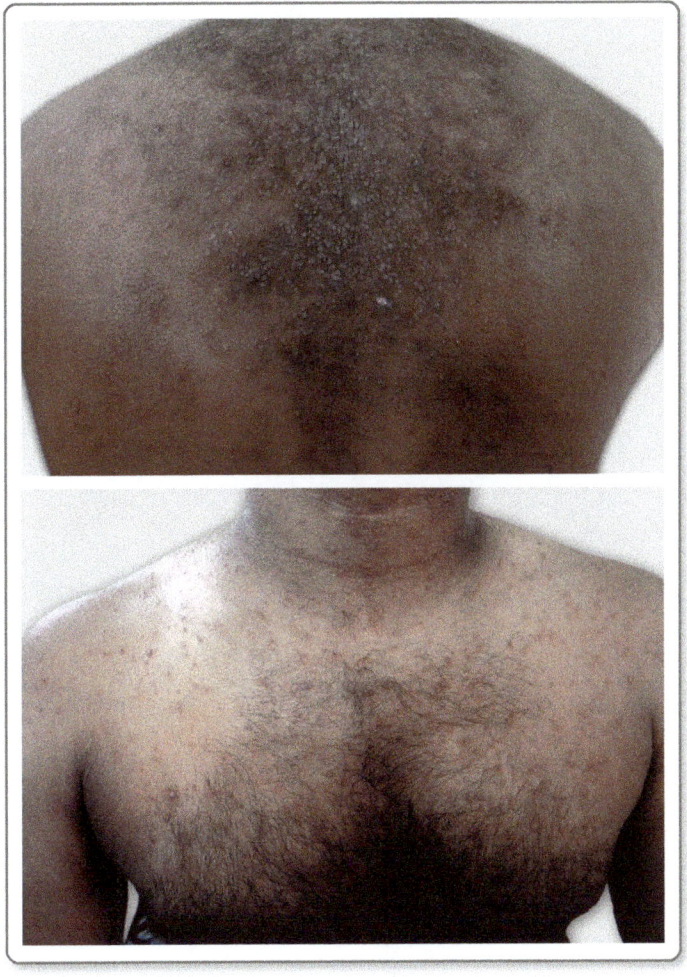

Q. What is the (i) diagnosis and (ii) management?

Answers

i. Seborrheic dermatitis
ii. Management:
    - Avoidance of oil/oily lotion
    - Oral tetracycline/doxycycline
    - Topical antifungal–steroid combination

Case 96

A 28-year-old lady had history of tick-bite followed by a progressively increased annular lesion with trail-like margin on left calf for last 6 weeks. She had no history of fever, arthralgia, cardiac, or neurological symptom.

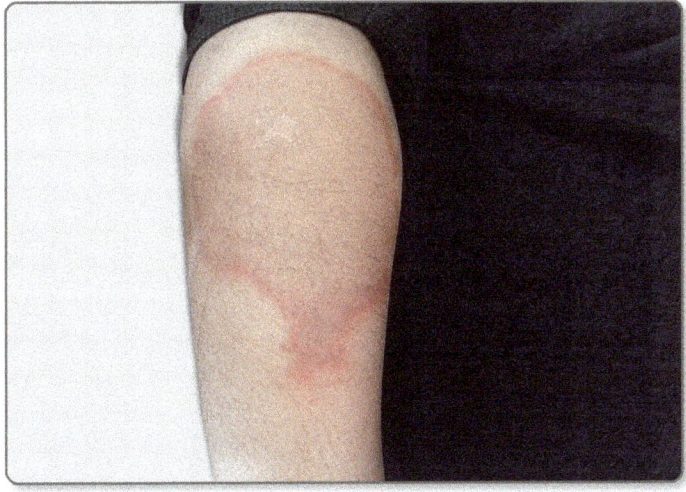

Q. What is the (i) diagnosis and (ii) management?

Answers

i. Erythema migrans
ii. Management:
   - Screening for systemic symptoms of Borreliosis
   - Oral doxycycline 100 mg twice daily for 3 weeks
     - Or oral erythromycin 250 mg four times daily for 3 weeks

Case 97

A 34-year-old female had erythematous pruritic eruption on face, neck, and forearms for last 5 months. Her submental area was not spared (white arrows). She had been contact with cement dust during her profession of construction supervisor.

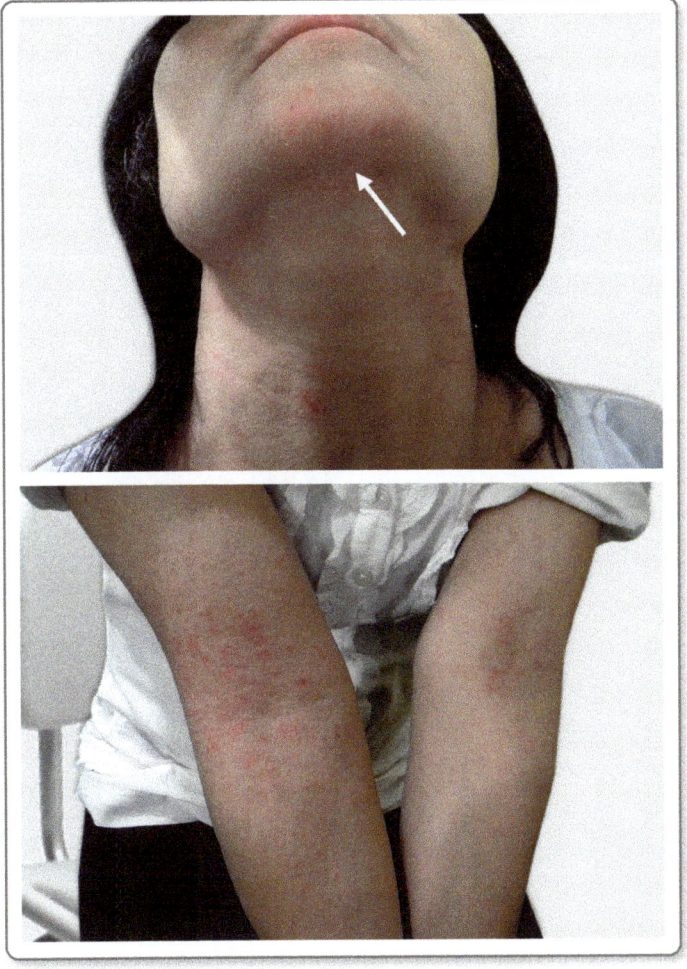

Q. What is the (i) diagnosis and (ii) management?

Answers

i. Airborne contact dermatitis to cement dust (potassium dichromate) [in photoallergic contact dermatitis (PACD) submental area is spared].
ii. Management:
   - To avoid cement dust as far as possible by using full sleeves, etc.
   - Topical low potent steroid or tacrolimus on face
   - Topical potent steroid on trunk and limbs
   - Antihistamines
   - Oral short course steroid, if refractory

Case 98

A 32-year-old male had sudden development of depigmented patch surrounding a pigmented mole during last 3 months.

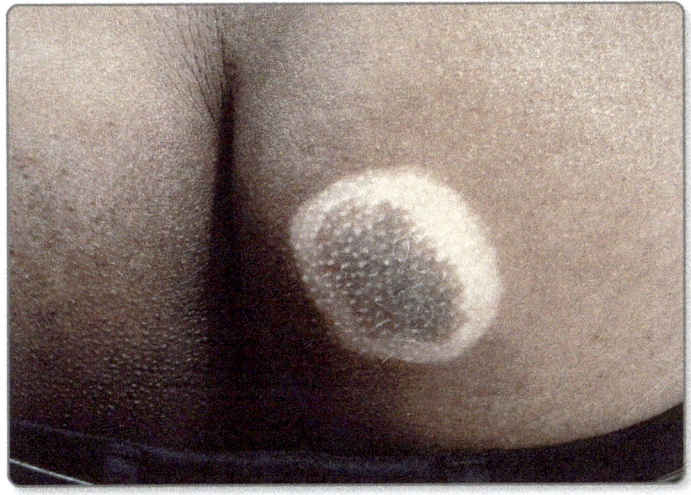

Q. What is the (i) diagnosis and (ii) management?

Answers

i. Halo nevus
ii. Management:
   - Topical tacrolimus 0.1% twice daily or topical steroid once daily
   - In refractory case, total excision of the mole

Case 99

A 49-year-old female had diffuse alopecia of scalp with frontal margin preserved for last 5 years.

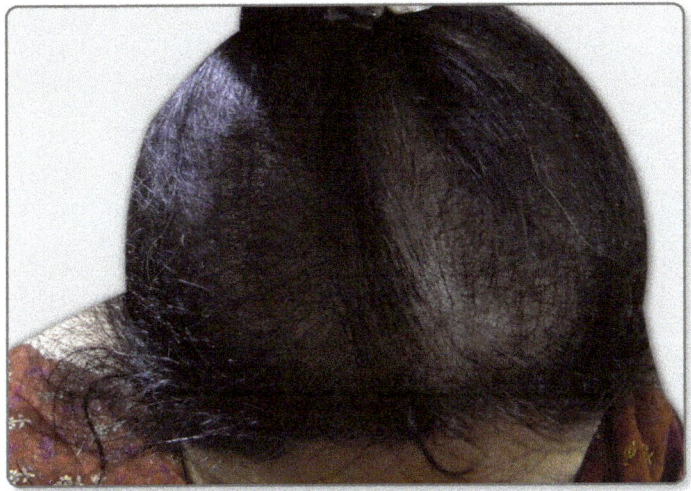

Q. What is the (i) diagnosis and (ii) management?

Answers

i. Female pattern hair loss (Ludwig type)
ii. Management:
   - Screening for hematological, gynecological, and endocrinological status
   - Topical minoxidil 2% lotion 1 mL twice daily for 6 months

Case 100

A 52-year-old female had asymptomatic pigmented macules and patches on lower legs and feet for last 2 years.

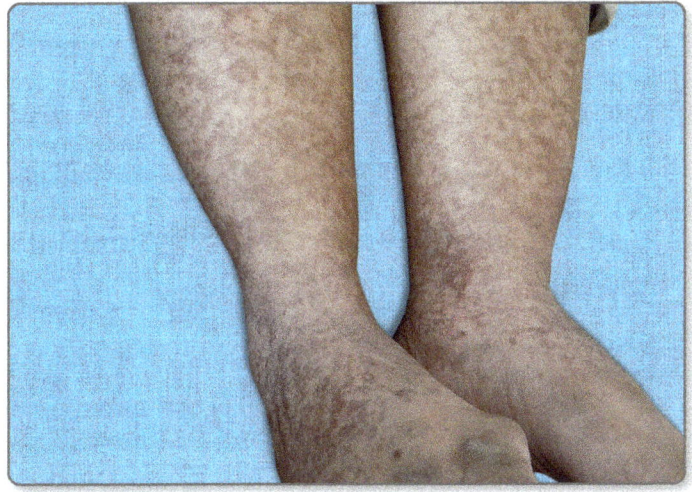

Q. What is the (i) diagnosis and (ii) management?

Answers

i. Pigmented purpuric dermatoses (PPD)
ii. Management:
   - To rule out underlying venous stasis
   - To avoid prolonged standing
   - To avoid calcium channel blockers
   - Potent topical steroids

Case 101

A 14-year-old male had chronic eczematous lesion on left foot for last 6 months. He had started the ailment after wearing a new "*chappal*".

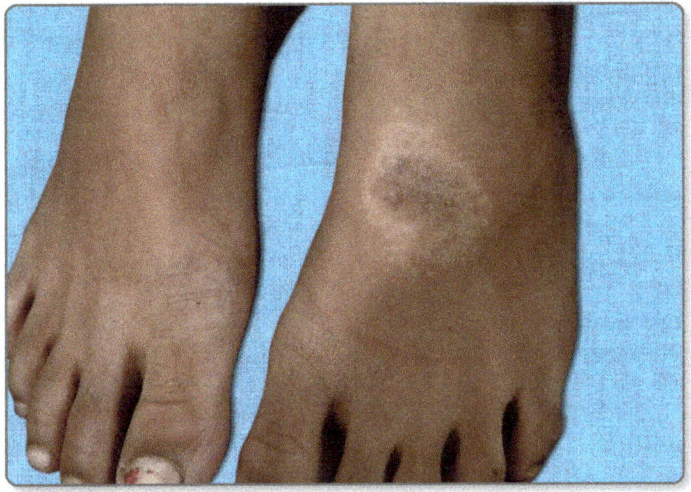

Q. What is the (i) diagnosis, (ii) management?

Answers

i. Allergic contact dermatitis from footwear (may be unilateral).
ii. Management:
    - Confirmation and detection of exact allergen of footwear by allergic patch test
    - Avoidance of relevant allergens
    - Topical corticosteroid

Case 102

A 13-year-old boy had recurrent pruritic vesicles on palm and feet for last 4 years.

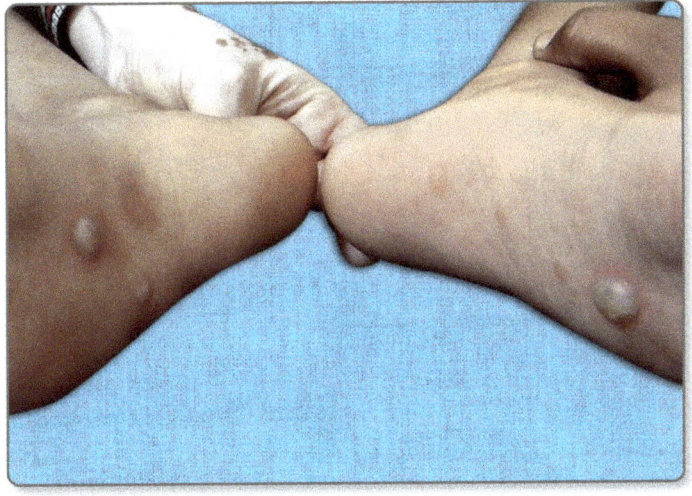

Q. What is the (i) diagnosis and (ii) management?

Answers

i. Vesicular dermatitis of hands and feet (pompholyx)
ii. Management:
    - To detect any associated fungal infection or eczematous lesions or septic focus inside body
    - To do allergic patch testing to detect the causative allergens if any
    - Topical corticosteroid
    - Oral antihistamines

Case 103

A 34-year-old male had recurrent intertriginous eruption on groin (black arrow) for last 5 years which mostly aggravated during winter. He had also thick hyperkeratotic lesions (white arrow) on knees and elbows.

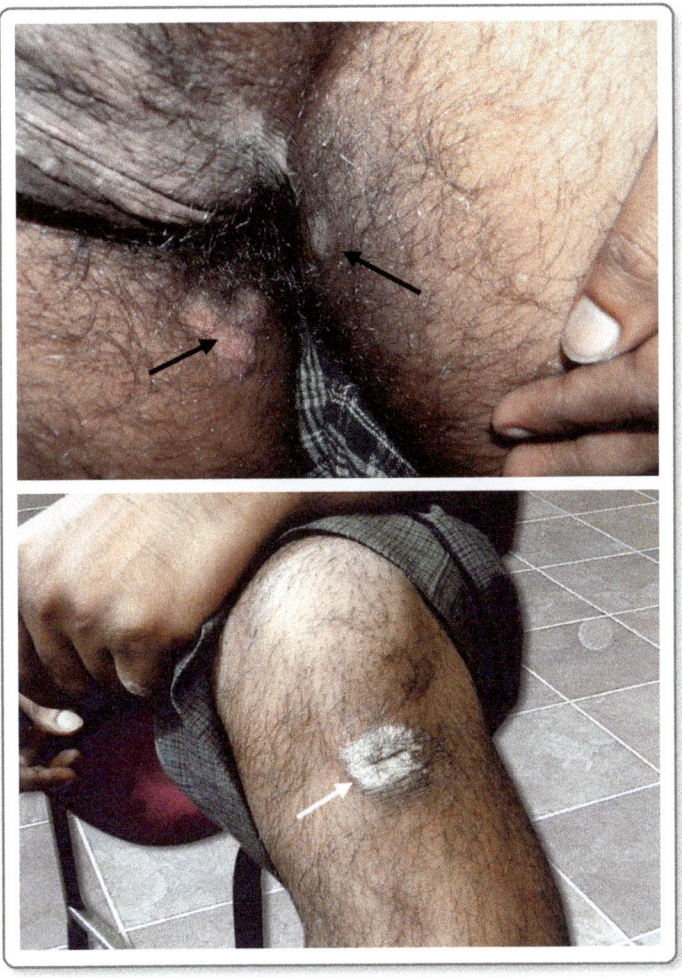

Q. What is the (i) diagnosis and (ii) management?

Answers

i. Flexural (inverse) psoriasis with chronic plaque psoriasis.
ii. Management:
    - Topical tacrolimus 0.3–0.1% or pimecrolimus 1% twice daily on groin patches.
    - Management of chronic plaque psoriasis as per body surface area (BSA) involvement.

Case 104

A 26-year-old female had chronic pruritic plaques for last 3 years. She had also oral lacy pattern of lesions for last 4 years.

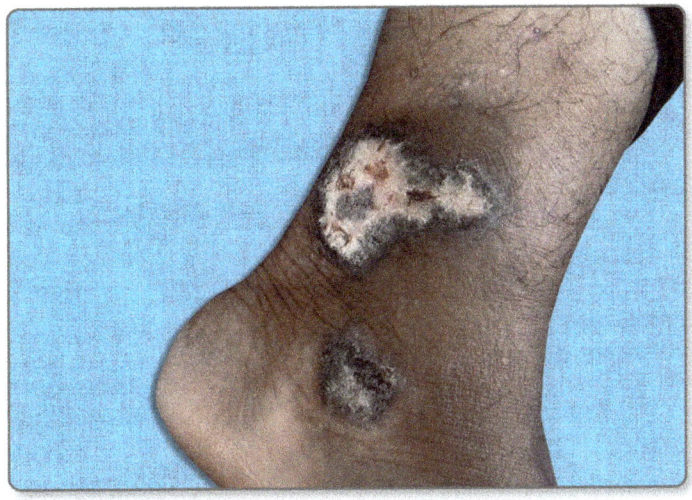

Q. What is the (i) diagnosis and (ii) management?

Answers

i. Lichen planus hypertrophicus
ii. Management:
   - Superpotent topical steroid by monitoring
   - Intralesional triamcinolone by expert dermatologist
   - Oral antihistamines

Case 105

A 41-year-old male had well-circumscribed hyperkeratotic lesions on feet for last 5 years mostly aggravating in winter. He had nail pitting and well-defined scaly plaques on scalp.

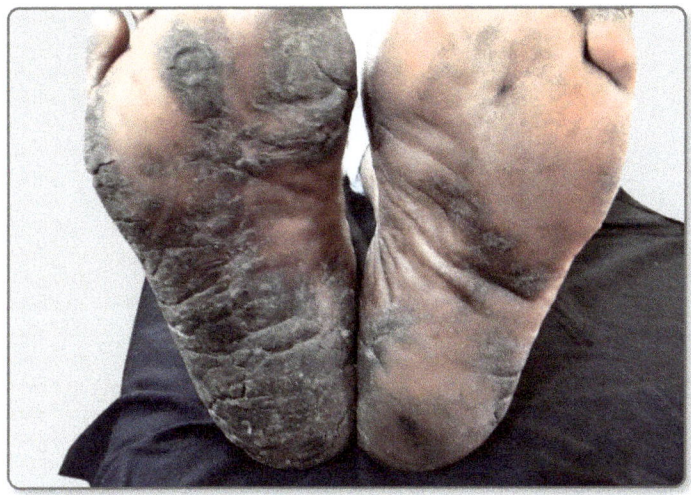

Q. What is the (i) diagnosis and (ii) management?

Answers

i. Plantar psoriasis
ii. Management:
   - Topical superpotent corticosteroid with or without 3% salicylic acid.
   - Topical tar or dithranol (short contact)
   - If refractory, PUVA or methotrexate or apremilast or acitretin under expert dermatologist.

Case 106

A 26-year-old male had sudden-onset maculopapular eruption on trunk, limbs and palms, and sole for last 5 days. He had history of oral amoxycillin 1 week back for throat infection.

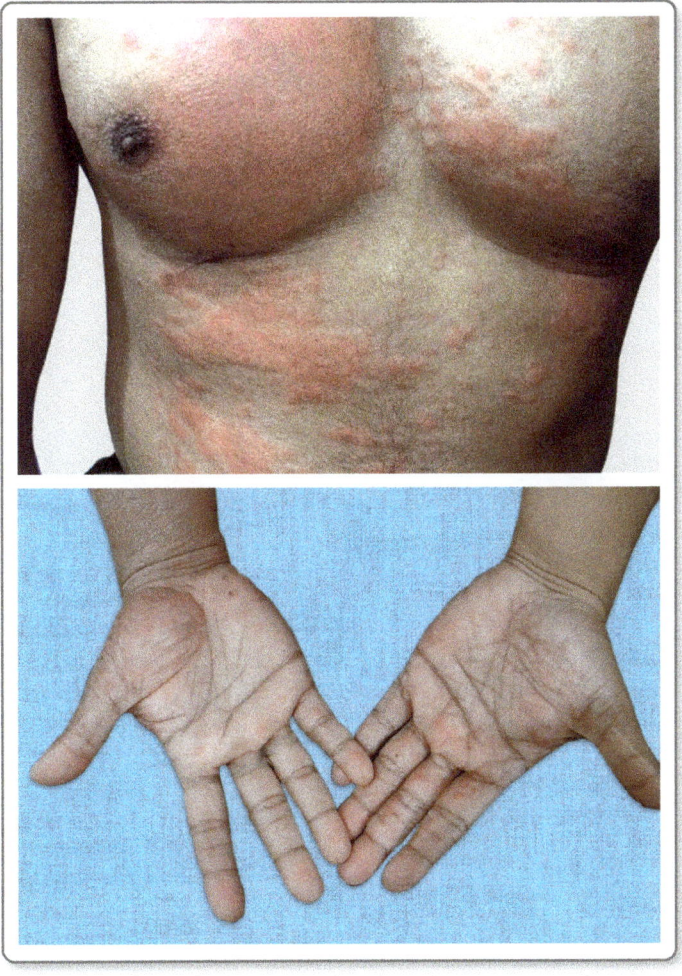

Q. What is the (i) diagnosis and (ii) management?

Answers

i. Adverse cutaneous drug eruption (maculopapular)
ii. Management:
   - Strict avoidance of relevant drugs and cross-reactants
   - Monitoring for systemic involvement
   - Topical corticosteroid lotion or cream
   - Oral antihistamines
   - Short course of oral steroids, if severe

Case 107

A 26-year-old lady developed acneiform eruption on lower face mostly along jaw lines along with excess terminal hairs on face for last 4 years. She had menstrual irregularities for last 5 years.

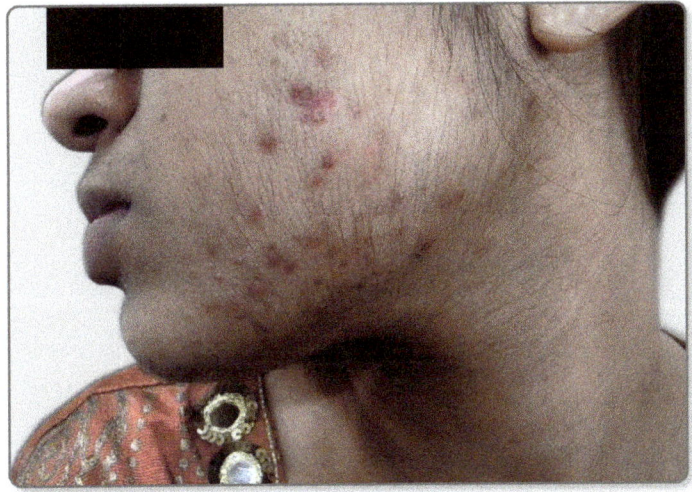

Q. What is the (i) diagnosis and (ii) management?

Answers

i. Acne and hirsutism probably due to polycystic ovarian diseases (PCOD)
ii. Management:
   - Referral to gynecologist
   - Topical clindamycin, benzoyl peroxide, and adapalene for acne
   - Topical eflornithine cream with or without laser for hirsutism

Case 108

A 68-year-old male had well-defined scaly erythematous plaques on different area of trunk (periumbilical, pubic area, etc.) and extensor surface of limbs. The scales were loose, white, and scraping the scales leads to bleeding (Auspitz sign positive).

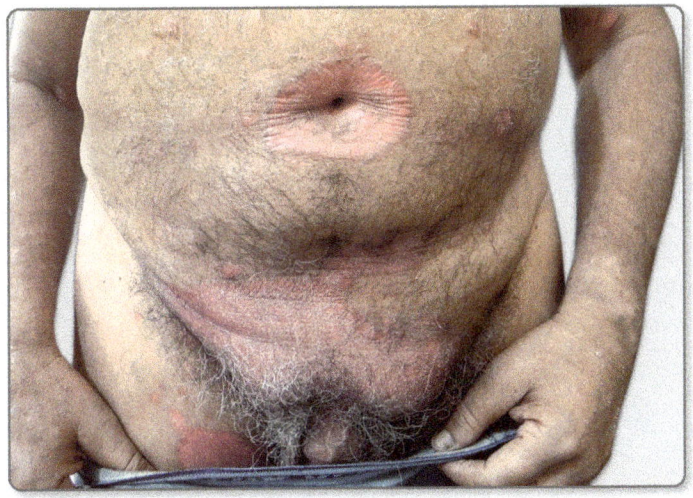

Q. What is the (i) diagnosis and (ii) management?

Answers

i. Psoriasis vulgaris (chronic plaque)
ii. Management:
  - Topical emollient
  - Topical low-potent steroid
  - UVB narrow band or PUVA
  - *If refractory*: Oral methotrexate or apremilast or biologics injection by screening and monitoring

Case 109

A 31-year-old male had warty lesion on glans (black arrow) for last 6 months. He had history of extramarital sexual exposure.

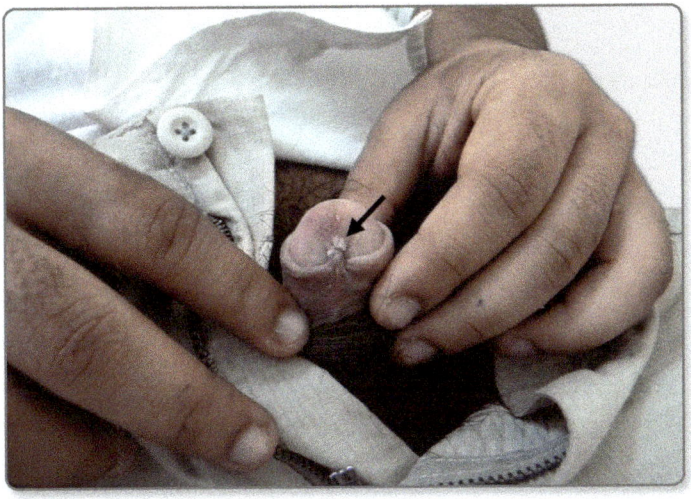

Q. What is the (i) diagnosis and (ii) management?

Answers

i. Condyloma acuminata
ii. Management:
   - Screening for other sexually transmitted diseases (STDs), especially HIV
   - Imiquimod 5% thrice in a week
   - Cryosurgery or electrosurgery under expert dermatologist

Case 110

A 31-year-old male had extensive hyperpigmented scaly lesions on trunk and limbs for last 2 months in summer. He had similar eruption in last 3 years during summer. On examination, the eruption had satellite lesions and perifollicular distribution.

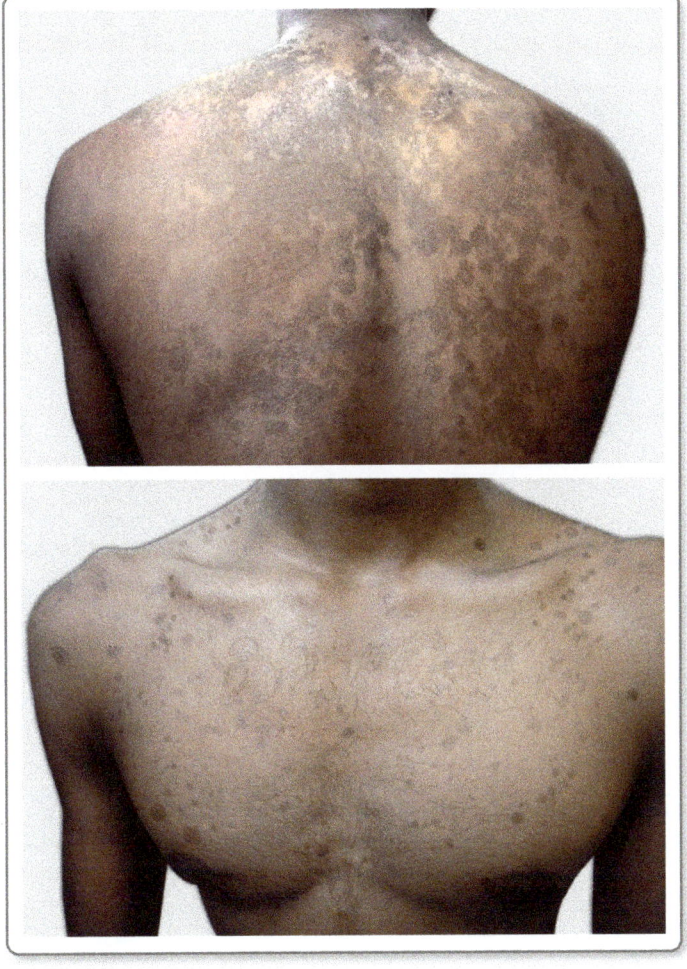

Q. What is the (i) diagnosis and (ii) management?

Answers

i. Pityriasis versicolor
ii. Management:
    - Topical 2% ketoconazole shampoo to apply for 5 minutes before bath for 3 consecutive days
    - *Oral antifungals*: Ketoconazole 200 mg daily for 7 days or itraconazole 100–200 mg twice daily for 7 days or fluconazole 400 mg stat.

Case 111

A 31-year-old lady had pruritic erythematous papular and pustular eruption on face for last 6 months. She had history of intermittent application of potent topical steroid for last 3 years.

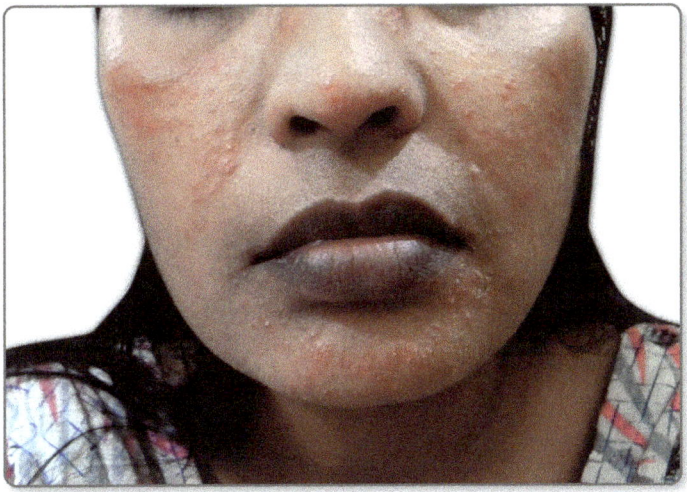

Q. What is the (i) diagnosis and (ii) management?

Answers

i. Iatrosacea due to topical steroid
ii. Management:
    - Topical low-potent steroid to be gradually tapered off and to be followed by: Topical tacrolimus 0.03–0.1% or pimecrolimus twice daily.
    - *If refractory*: Oral tetracycline, doxycycline, or minocycline

Case 112

A 36-year-old male had recurrent painful boils-like eruption (black arrow) on scalp for last 2 years.

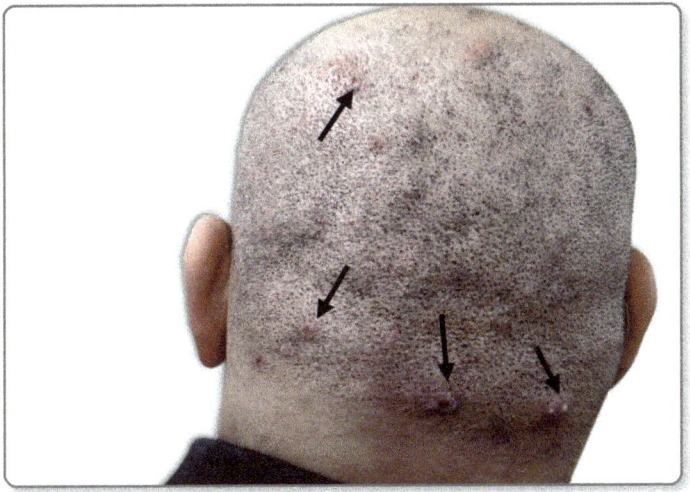

Q. What is the (i) diagnosis and (ii) management?

Answers

i. Folliculitis decalvans
ii. Management:
   - Oral tetracycline or doxycycline or minocycline for long-term
   - Topical ozenoxacin, mupirocin, or fusidic acid
   - Povidone iodine shampoo

Case 113

A 64-year-old male had gradual onset bullous eruption which were tense and hemorrhagic (black arrow) during last 6 months. He had no oral mucosal lesion.

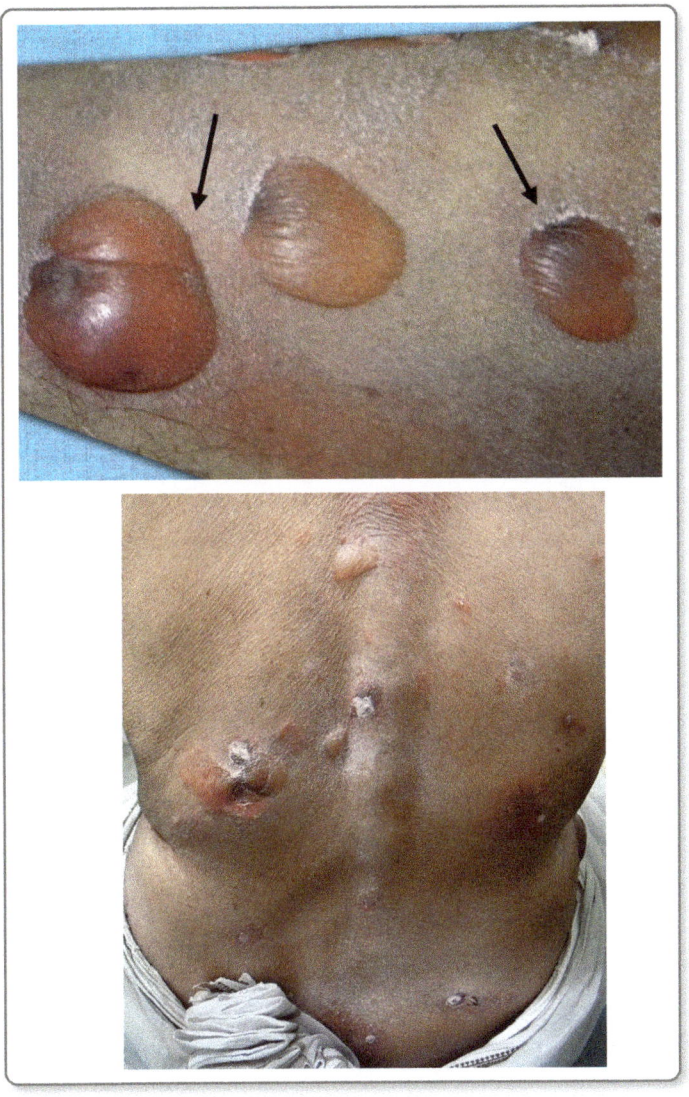

Q. What is the (i) diagnosis and (ii) management?

Answers

i. Bullous pemphigoid
ii. Management:
   - Confirmation of diagnosis by skin biopsy
   - Avoidance of gliptin (antidiabetic) if any
   - Oral corticosteroid and adjuvant (azathioprine, mycophenolate mofetil, etc.) under expert dermatologist by strict monitoring

Case 114

A 65-year-old lady had sudden-onset pain in left ear and left side of face followed by grouped vesicular eruption in dermatomal distribution (black arrow) and external ear (blue arrow) for last 3 days.

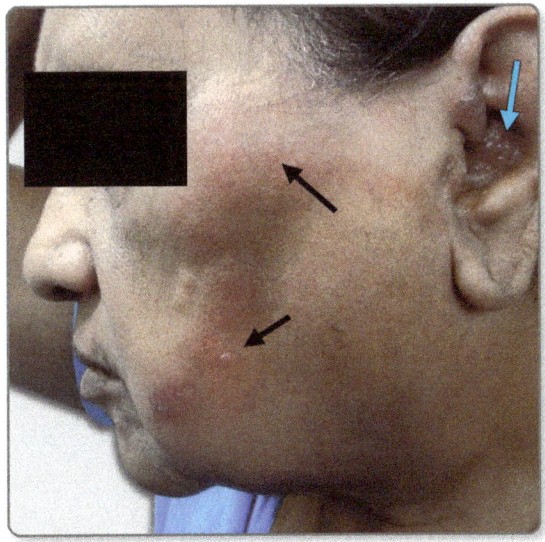

Q. What is the (i) diagnosis and (ii) management?

Answers

i. Herpes zoster oticus (Ramsay Hunt syndrome)
ii. Management:
   - Referral to ENT surgeon to manage for facial palsy, if any
   - Oral valacyclovir 1,000 mg thrice daily or acyclovir 800 mg five times daily or famciclovir 500 mg thrice daily for 7 days.

Case 115

A 23-year-old male had multiple painful hard noduloulcerative lesions on glans and prepuce for last 1 week. He had associated painful lymphadenopathy. He had history of exposure to a sexual worker.

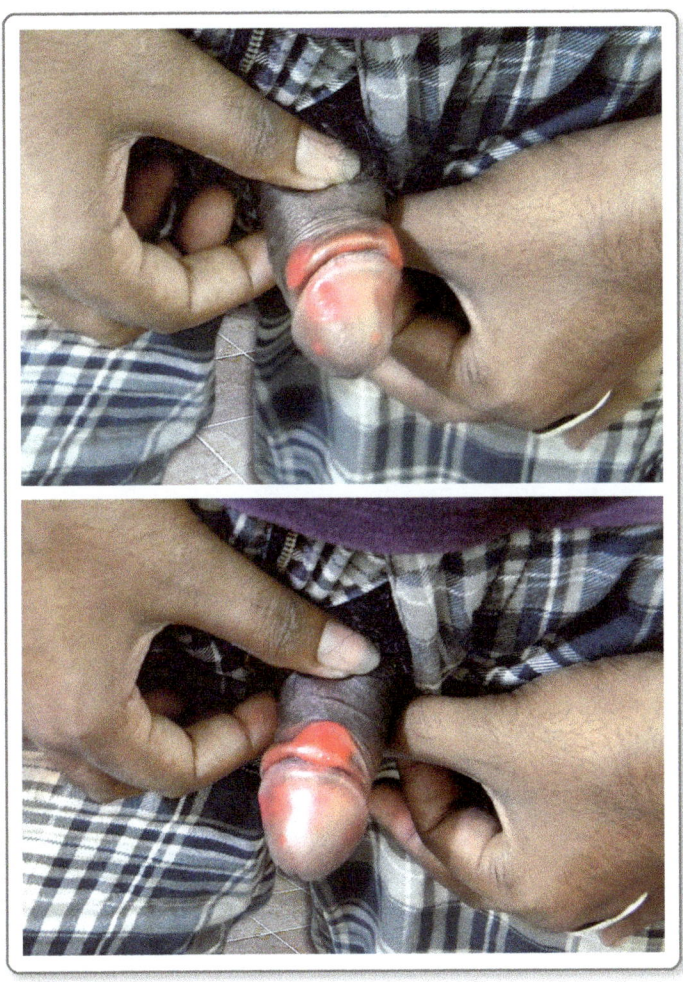

Q. What is the (i) diagnosis and (ii) management?

Answers

i. Chancroid
ii. Management:
   - Screening for other STDs, especially HIV
   - Azithromycin 1 g single dose
     Or ceftriaxone 250 mg IM single dose
     Or ciprofloxacin 500 mg BID for 3 days
     Or erythromycin 500 mg four times daily for 7 days

Case 116

A 49-year-old male had coppery colored hypoesthetic patches on right elbow and right side of abdomen (black arrows) for last 6 months. Right radial nerve was thickened but not tender.

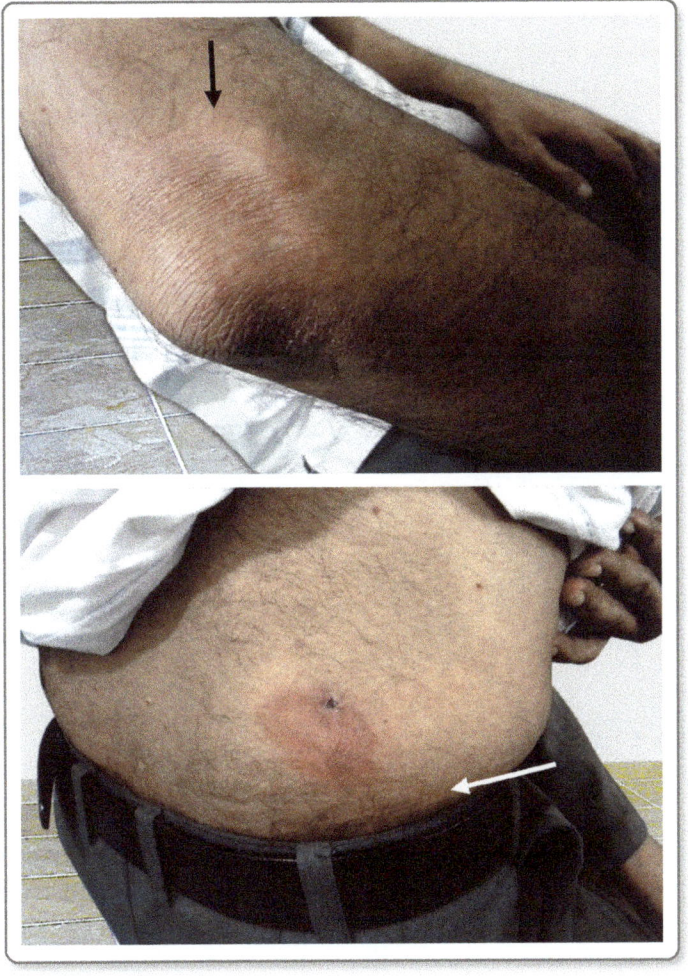

Q. What is the (i) diagnosis and (ii) management?

Answers

i. Hanseniasis [paucibacillary: borderline tuberculoid (BT)]
ii. Management:
    - Dapsone 100 mg daily
    - Rifampicin 600 mg orally once in empty stomach (supervised)

Case 117

A 26-year-old lady had generalized pustular eruption (black arrow) and lake of pus (blue arrow) with fever for last 3 months. She had previous history of psoriasis vulgaris and been treated with oral corticosteroids.

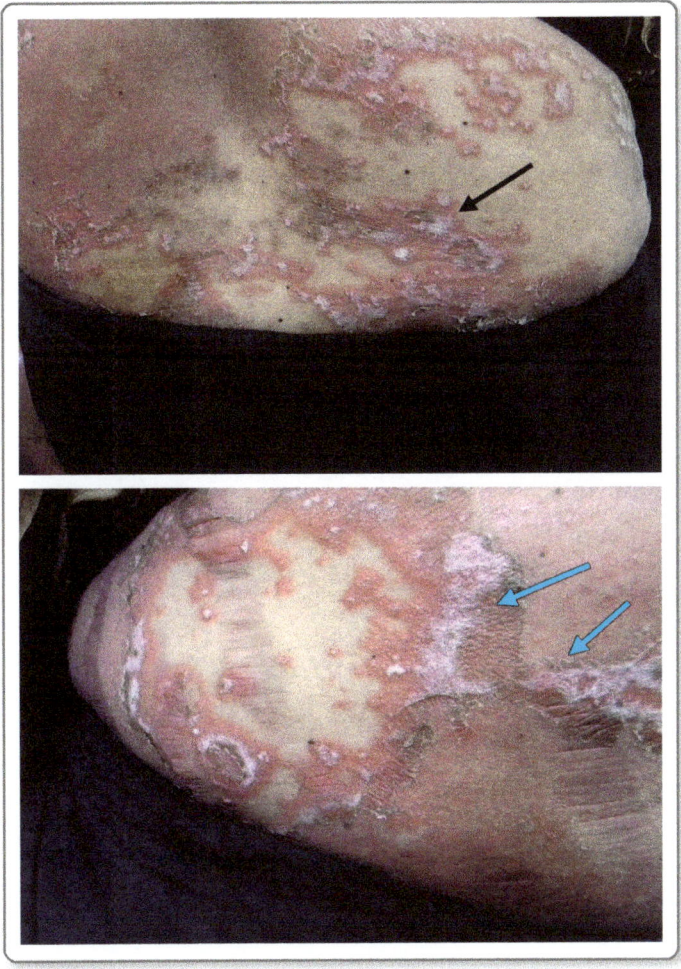

Q. What is the (i) diagnosis and (ii) management?

Answers

i. Pustular psoriasis
ii. Management:
- ➤ Admission under dermatologist and internist
- ➤ Oral cyclosporine under expert dermatologist

Case 118

A 31-year-old lady had recurrent acneiform eruption around mouth for last 8 months. She had history of application of topical corticosteroid and lot of cosmetics.

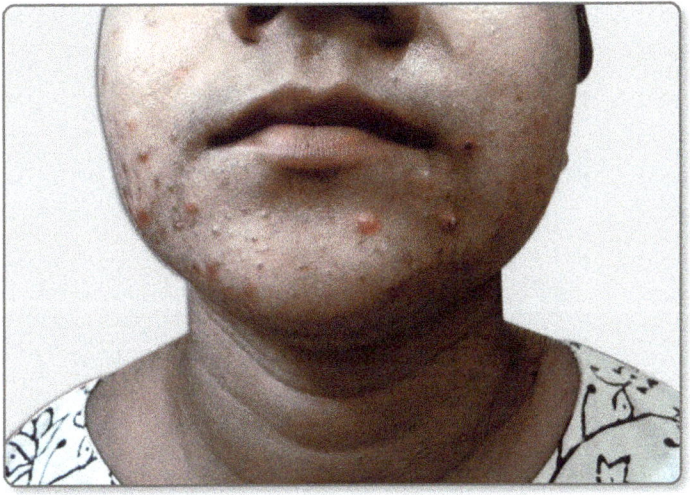

Q. What is the (i) diagnosis and (ii) management?

Answers

i. Perioral dermatitis
ii. Management:
   - Oral tetracycline or doxycycline
   - Topical clindamycin or benzoyl peroxide

Case 119

A 35-year-old male had multiple umbilicated papules around genitalia for last 5 months. He had extramarital partner.

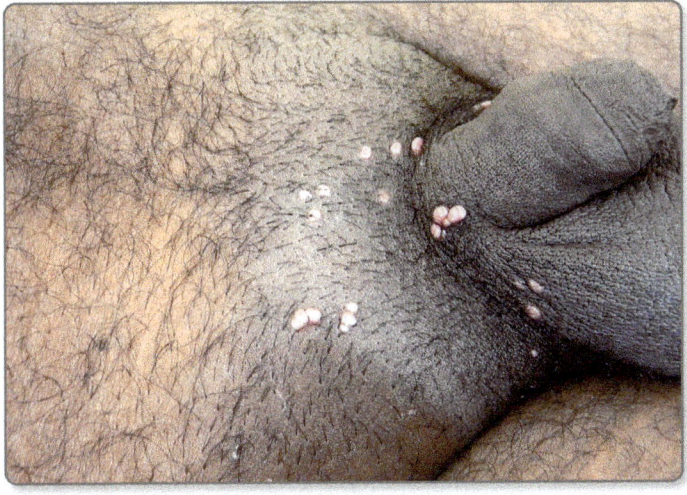

Q. What is the (i) diagnosis and (ii) management?

Answers

i. Molluscum contagiosum (perigenital)
ii. Management:
   - Screening for other STDs, especially HIV
   - Extraction and chemical cautery
     Or electrosurgery
     Or cryosurgery

Case 120

A 23-year-old female had multiple discharging ulcers with underlying lymphadenopathy on left side of neck for last 1 year. She had history of low-grade fever, cough, night sweating, and loss of weight.

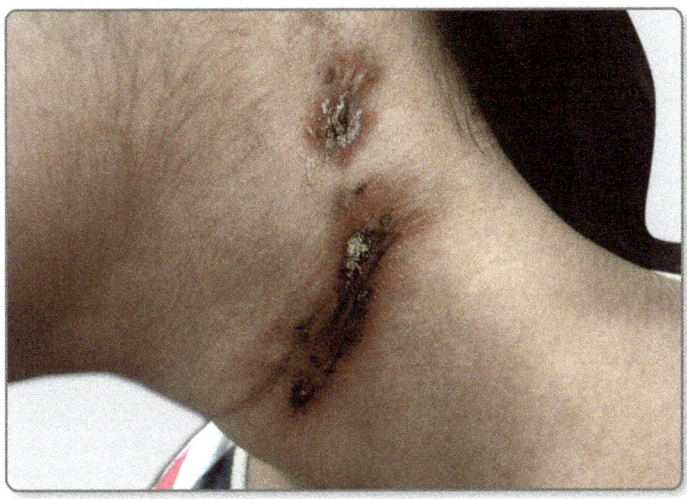

Q. What is the (i) diagnosis and (ii) management?

Answers

i. Scrofuloderma
ii. Management:
   - Referral to tuberculosis specialist and surgeon
   - Confirmation of diagnosis
   - Full antituberculous regimen under tuberculosis specialist

Case 121

A 4-month-old female infant had extensive eczematous eruption on extensor aspect of limbs, face, and trunk for last 1 month. She had history of bronchial spasm and family history of asthma and eczema.

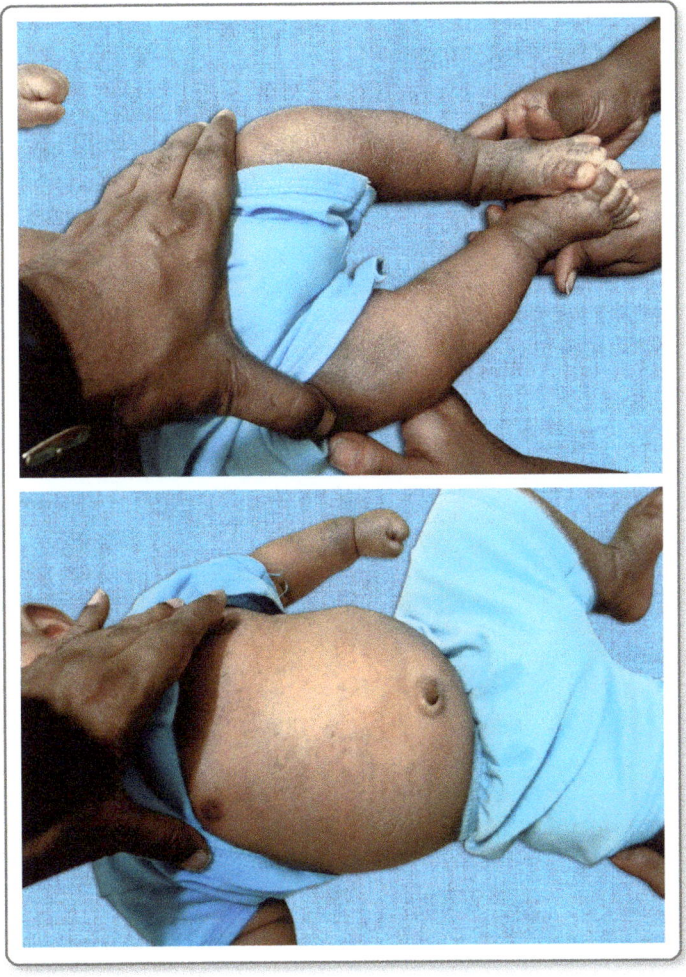

Q. What is the (i) diagnosis and (ii) management?

Answers

i. Atopic dermatitis (*in infants extensor aspect involved compared to flexural involvement in older children*)
ii. Management:
    - Topical emollients
    - Low-potent topical steroid
    - Avoidance of atopic triggers

Case 122

A 52-year-old female had extensive pruritic eruption with complaints of some insects always crawling on her skin for last 3 years. She brought some dead insect-like objects in a plastic container. She expressed history of disharmony with her daughter-in-law.

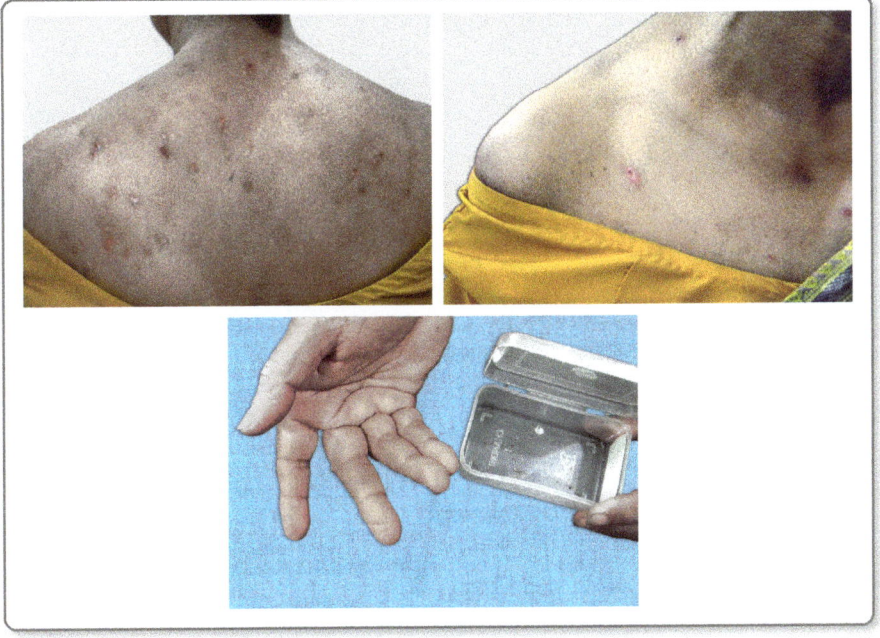

Q. What is the (i) diagnosis and (ii) management?

Answers

i. Delusion of parasitosis
ii. Management:
- Referral to psychiatrist
- Topical calamine to relieve itching

Case 123

A 24-year-old female had malar flush, photosensitivity, oral ulceration on hard palate, skin eruption on photo-exposed skin along with fever and arthralgia for last 1 year.

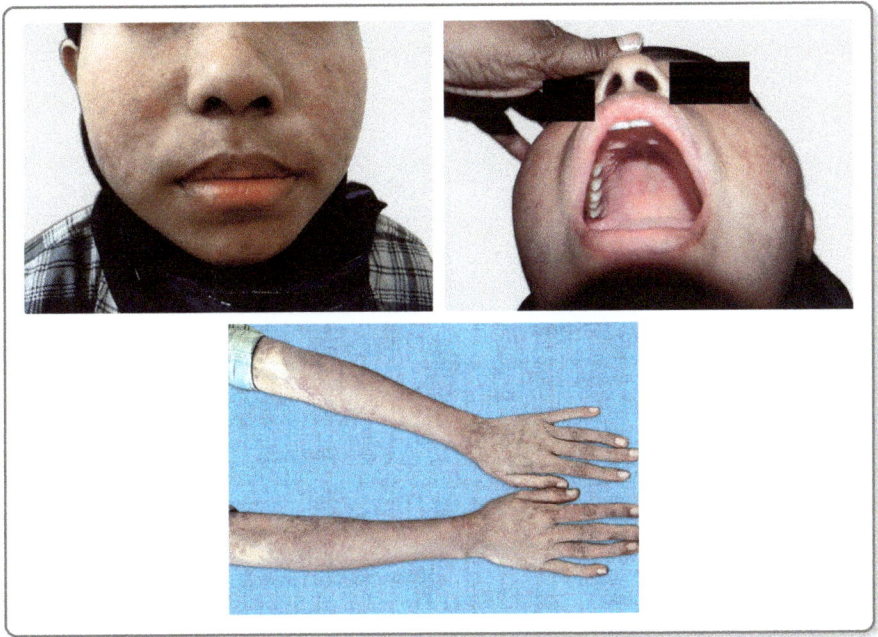

Q. What is the (i) diagnosis and (ii) management?

Answers

i. Systemic lupus erythematosus
ii. Management:
   - Referral to rheumatologist
   - Strict avoidance of day light
   - Oral hydroxychloroquine 200–400 mg by eye monitoring

Case 124

A 36-year-old male had swelling of left leg (unilaterally) with multiple discharging sinuses (black arrows) liberating pus-containing granules for last 10 years. On palpation, the affected area was not tender.

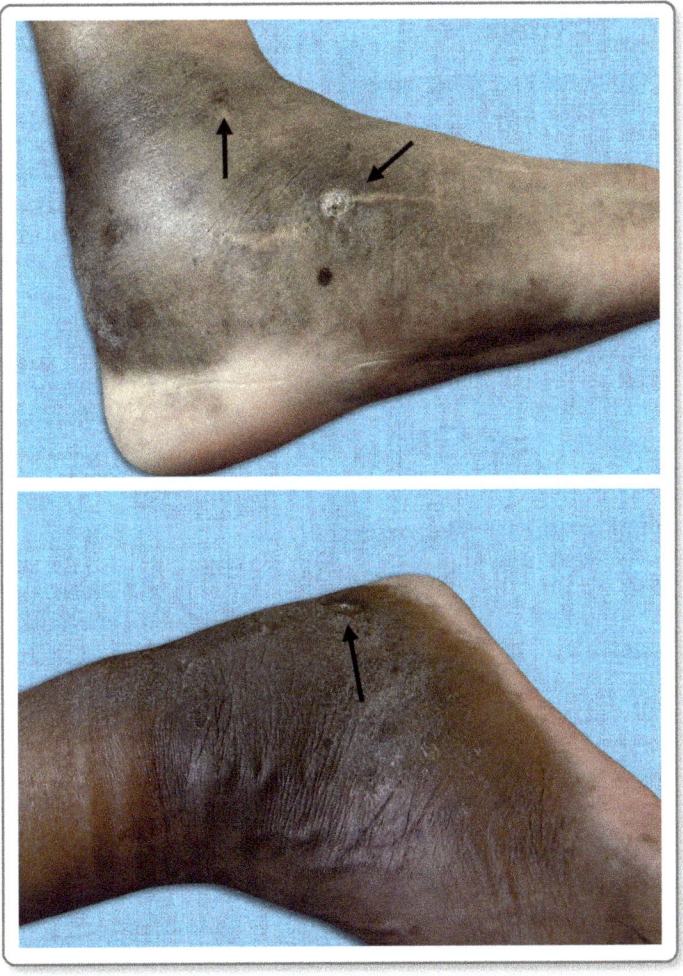

Q. What is the (i) diagnosis and (ii) management?

Answers

i. Mycetoma
ii. Management:
   - Confirmation of diagnosis and identification of etiological agents (actinomycetoma or eumycetoma, i.e., true fungi)
   - *Actinomycetoma*: Streptomycin or rifampicin with either cotrimoxazole or dapsone
   - *Eumycetoma*: Ketoconazole or itraconazole

Case 125

A 28-year-old primigravida at 28 weeks of gestation had itchy papules, wheals, and plaques on her abdomen especially on striae.

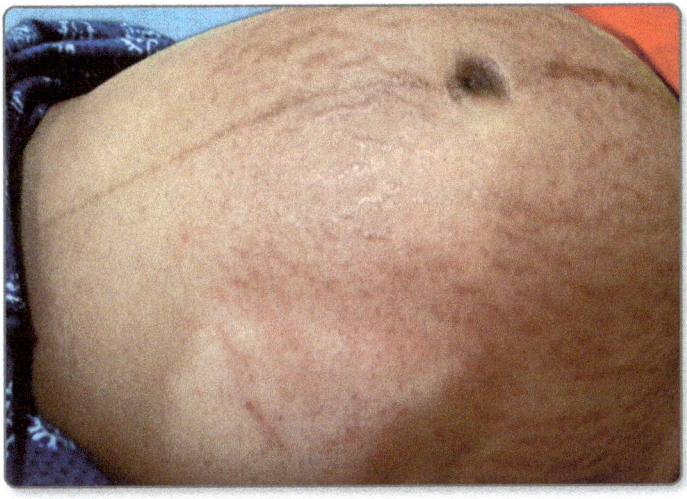

Q. What is the (i) diagnosis and (ii) management?

Answers

i. Polymorphic eruption of pregnancy
ii. Management:
   - Topical corticosteroid
   - Antihistamines (Loratadine)

Case 126

A 34-year-old lady had tiny pigmented macules (white arrows) on face for last 15 years aggravating after sun exposure. She had similar ailment in her mother.

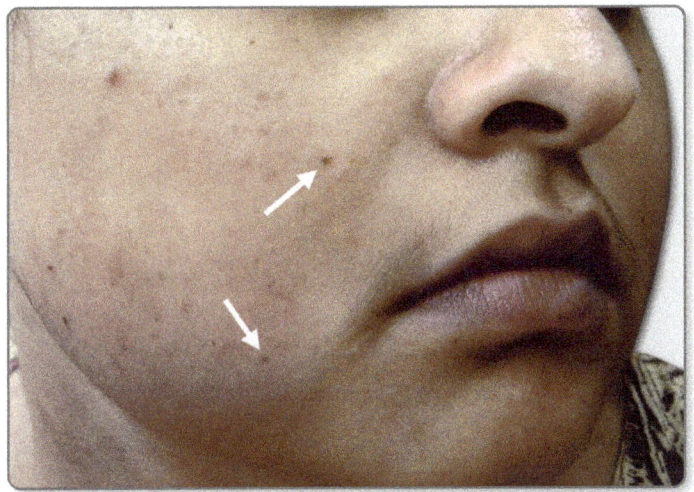

Q. What is the (i) diagnosis and (ii) management?

Answers

i. Freckles
ii. Management:
  - Avoidance of daylight by sunscreen, etc.
  - Prognosis (incurable nature) to be explained.

Case 127

A 54-year-old male had hyperkeratotic palms and soles for last 10 years with some warty lesions (black arrow). He had also dewdrops like hyper- and hypopigmentation over trunk. He had history of ingestion of tubewell water for last 15 years.

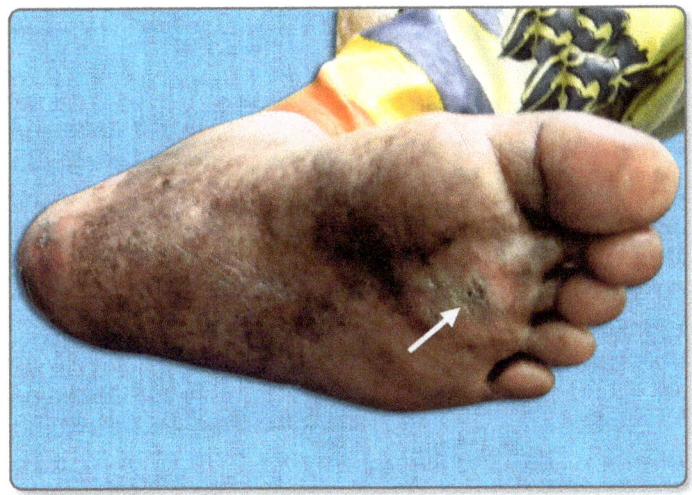

Q. What is the (i) diagnosis and (ii) management?

Answers

i. Arsenic keratosis
ii. Management:
    - Avoidance of tubewell water
    - Avoid other carcinogens (smoking, sun exposure, etc.)
    - Biopsy from the warty lesions to exclude malignancy.

Case 128

A 24-year-old female had recurrent small scaly plaques (black arrow) on limbs and trunk for last 1 year.

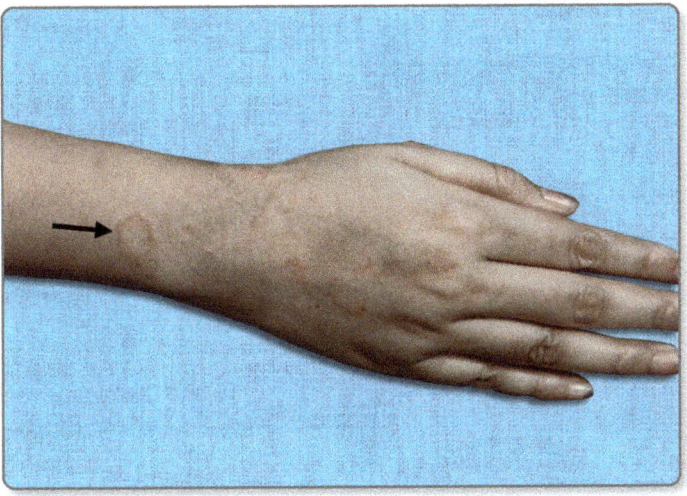

Q. What is the (i) diagnosis and (ii) management?

Answers

i. Small plaque parapsoriasis
ii. Management:
   - Topical steroid
   - UVB therapy/PUVA therapy

Case 129

A 29-year-old male had itchy papules on glans, shaft of the penis for last 2 months. He had history of extramarital exposure.

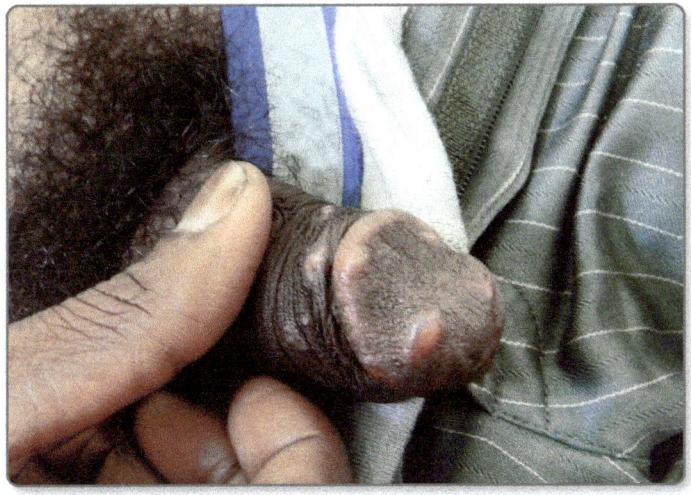

Q. What is the (i) diagnosis and (ii) management?

Answers

i. Scabies (sexually acquired)
ii. Management:
   - Exclusion of other STDs by proper screening
   - Permethrin 5% to apply from neck to feet for 1 night (to repeat once next week)

Case 130

A 21-year-old male had soft swelling one side of left great toe nail for last 3 months which used to bleed often. He had history of trauma 6 months back on that site.

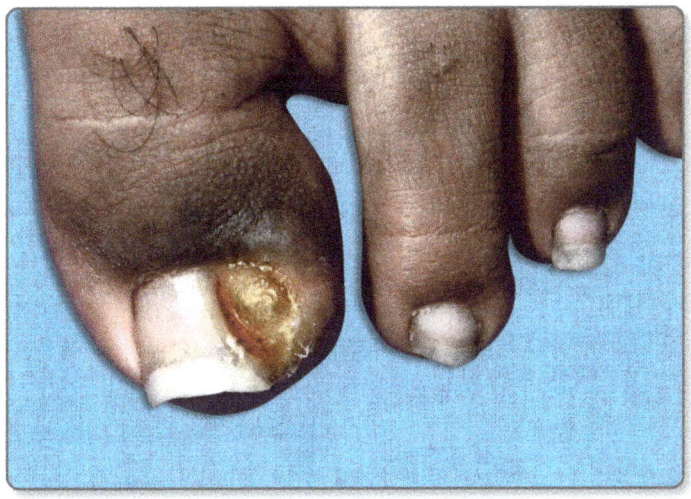

Q. What is the (i) diagnosis and (ii) management?

Answers

i. Granuloma pyogenicum
ii. Management:
   - Control of infection
   - Chemical cautery or electrocautery or cryotherapy

Case 131

A 26-year-old male recurrent painful chord-like swelling (black arrow) on legs for last 1 year.

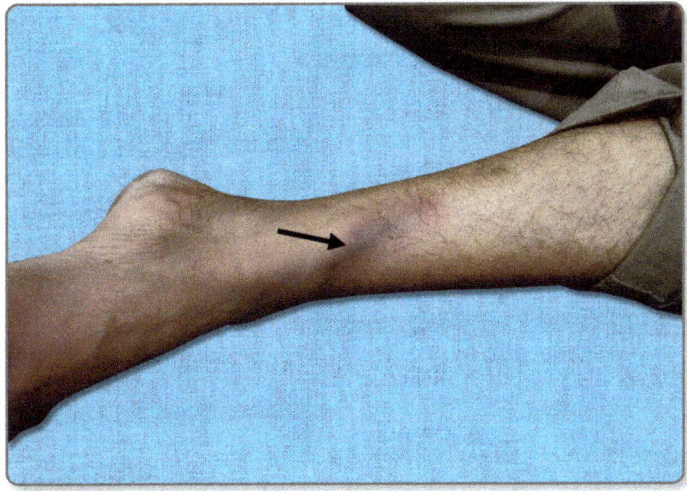

Q. What is the (i) diagnosis and (ii) management?

Answers

i. Recurrent thrombophlebitis
ii. Management:
   - Systemic antibiotics
   - To search any underlying diseases such as pancreatic carcinoma, tuberculosis, etc.

Case 132

A 59-year-old female had recurrent reddish swelling on both eyelids for last 1 year. She had history of taking angiotensin-converting enzyme (ACE) inhibitor as antihypertensive for last 2 years.

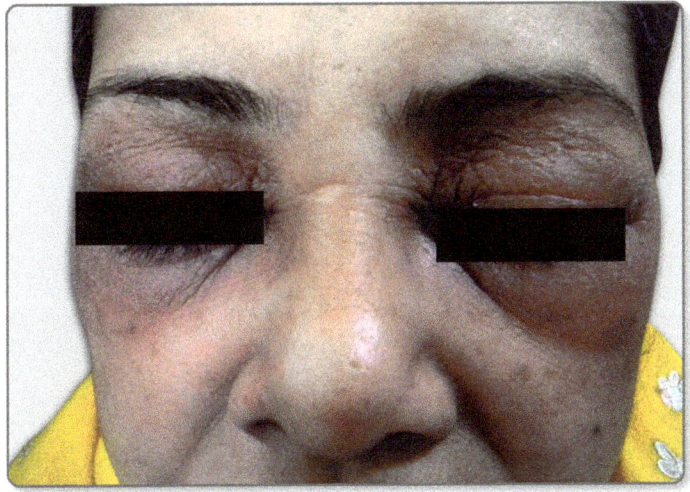

Q. What is the (i) diagnosis and (ii) management?

Answers

i. Acquired angioedema (due to ACE inhibitor)
ii. Management:
   - Avoidance of ACE inhibitors and also angiotensin-receptor blocking agents (sartan group)
   - Oral antihistaminic
   - Anti-bradykinin agent

Case 133

A 43-year-old male had oral erosion, generalized skin eruption (mostly maculopapular) for last 3 weeks with fever. His liver enzymes were quite high. He had history of taking allopurinol for last 2 months for hyperuricemia.

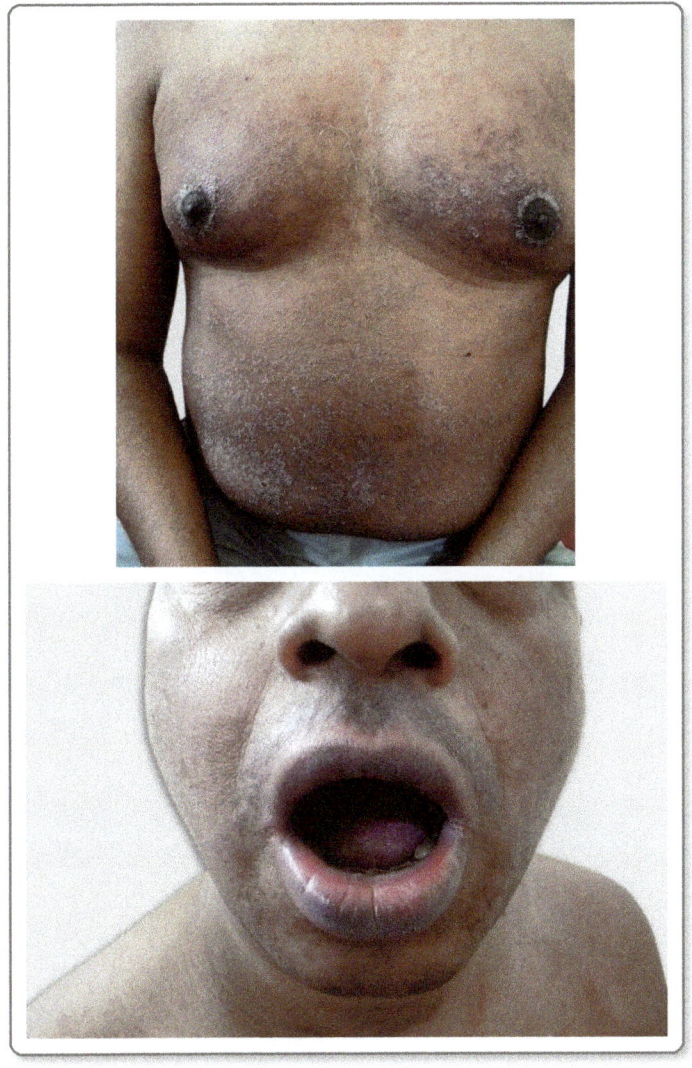

Q. What is the (i) diagnosis and (ii) management?

Answers

i. Drug hypersensitivity syndrome (DHS) (due to allopurinol)
ii. Management:
   - Immediate withdrawal of allopurinol
   - Admission under dermatologist and internist
   - Screening, monitoring, and supporting treatment of systemic involvement
   - Oral corticosteroid for long term by gradual tapering and monitoring

Case 134

A 64-year-old male had chronic dry eczematous lesions on lower legs for last 6 months being aggravated in winter.

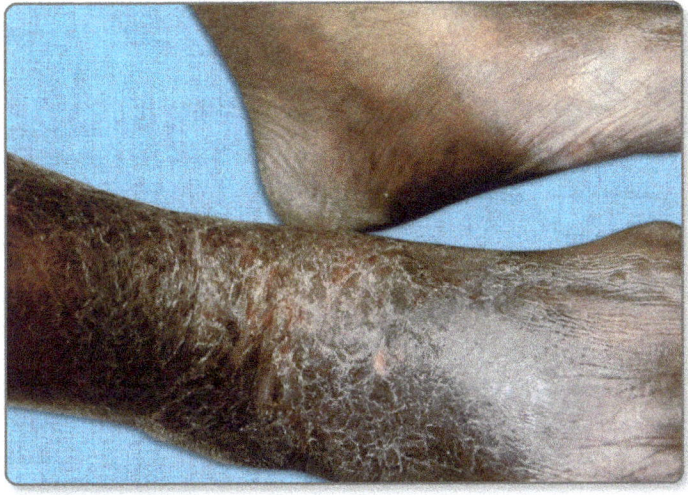

Q. What is the (i) diagnosis and (ii) management?

Answers

i. Asteatotic eczema
ii. Management:
   - Avoidance of soap
   - Screening for diabetes and hypothyroid
   - Topical emollient (containing urea, etc.)
   - Topical steroid in ointment for brief period
   - Oral antihistamines

Case 135

A 45-year-old female had swelling, puffiness, and nodules on ear lobules, face, and different area of trunk. The lesions were juicy, shiny, and soft.

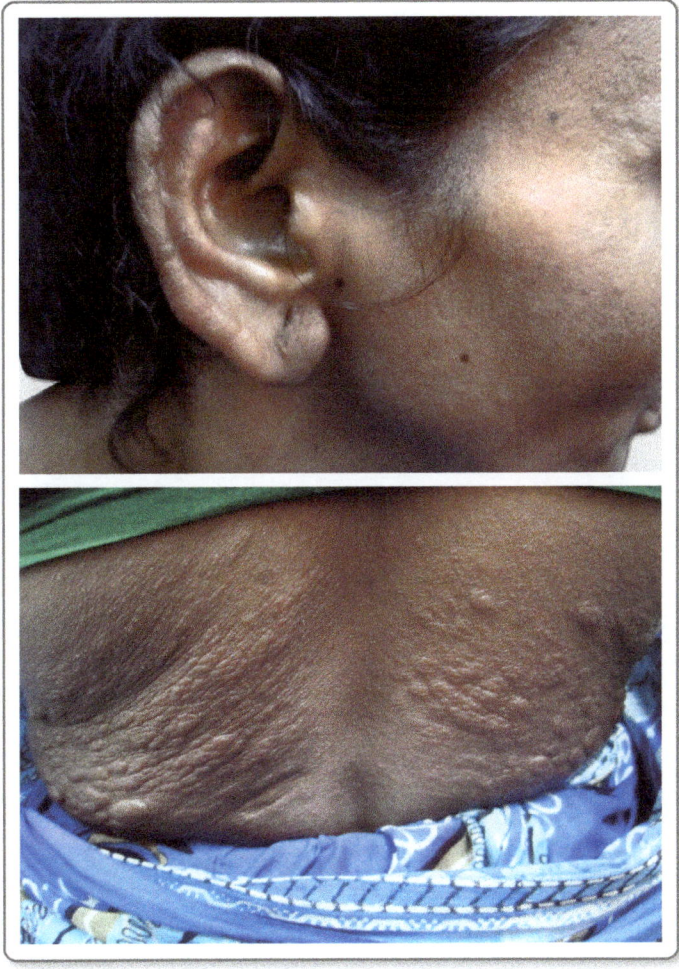

Q. What is the (i) diagnosis and (ii) management?

Answers

i. Lepromatous leprosy
ii. Management:
- Dapsone 100 mg daily
- Clofazimine 100 mg on alternate day, and 300 mg once monthly
- Rifampicin 600 mg once monthly in empty stomach (supervised)

Case 136

A 47-year-old female had multiple skin-colored nodules on axillae and neck for last 3 years. She had history of diabetes for last 10 years.

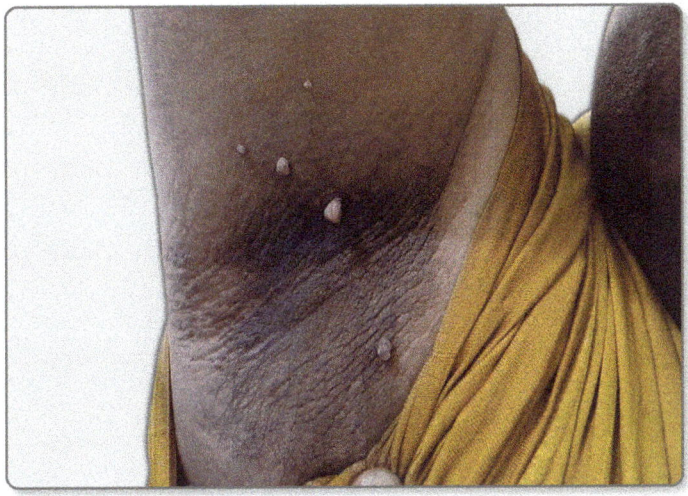

Q. What is the (i) diagnosis and (ii) management?

Answers

i. Acrochordon (skin tags)
ii. Management:
- Control of diabetes
- Electrocautery or cryotherapy

Case 137

A 21-year-old female had highly pruritic hyperkeratotic papules or nodules on limbs and trunk for last 2 years.

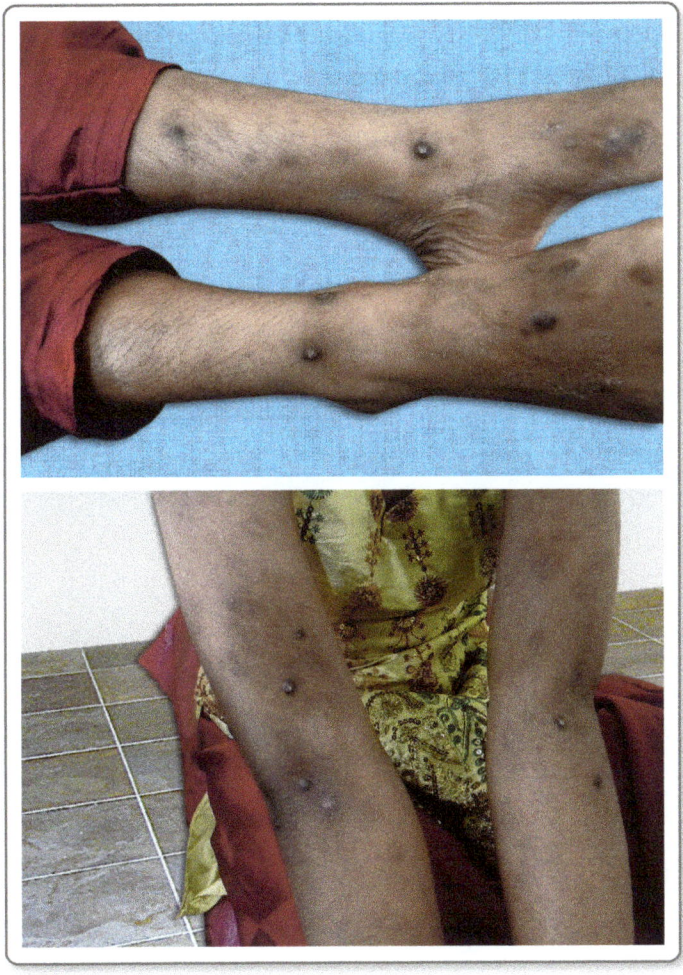

Q. What is the (i) diagnosis and (ii) management?

Answers

i. Prurigo nodularis
ii. Management:
   - Topical superpotent corticosteroid
   - Oral antihistaminic

Case 138

An 18-year-old male had linear depressed pigmented lesion (black arrow) on central forehead for last 3 years.

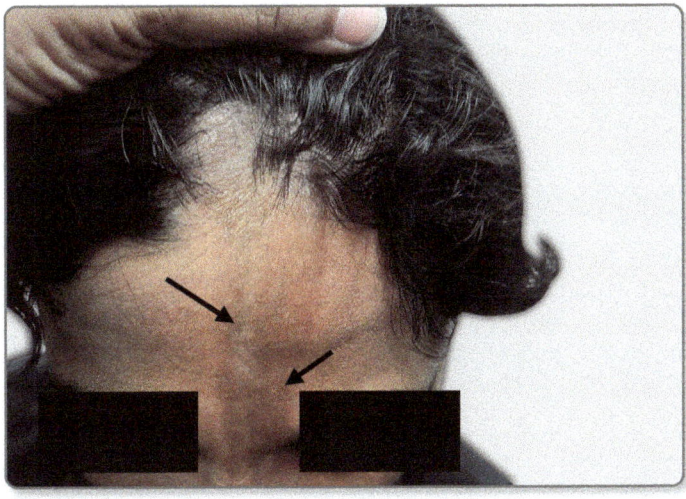

Q. What is the (i) diagnosis and (ii) management?

Answers

i. Linear morphea (localized scleroderma)
ii. Management:
   - Topical vitamin D analog
   - Topical mid-potent steroid

Case 139

A 10-year-old boy had recurrent itchy eczematous lesions on limbs and trunk predominately affecting flexors since last 5 years. He had also history of bronchial asthma.

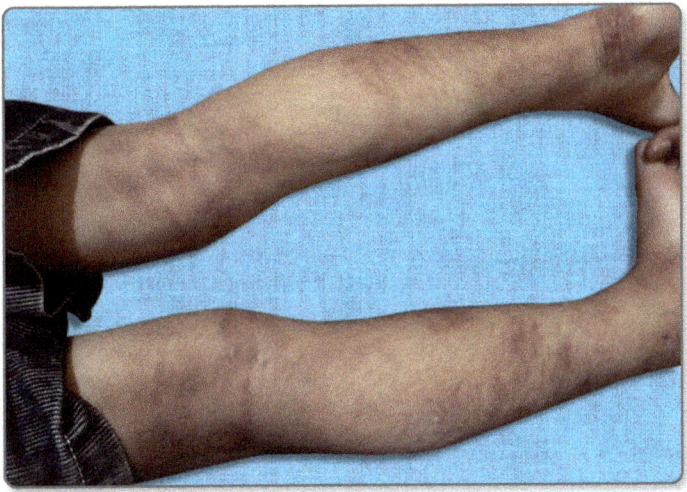

Q. What is the (i) diagnosis and (ii) management?

Answers

i. Atopic dermatitis
ii. Management:
   - Avoidance of triggering factors (dust mite, pollens, etc.)
   - Topical emollients liberally
   - Topical low-potent steroid or tacrolimus/pimecrolimus or crisaborole
   - Oral antihistamines

Case 140

A 51-year-old male had pruritic hives mostly in linear configuration especially after stroking.

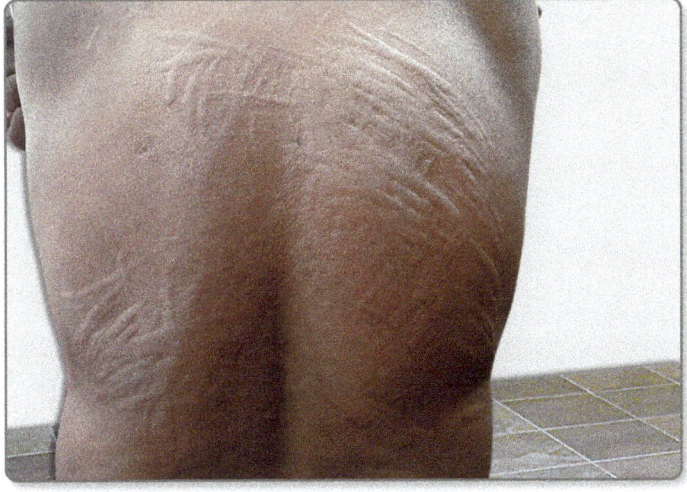

Q. What is the (i) diagnosis and (ii) management?

Answers

i. Dermographism (symptomatic)
ii. Management:
   - Avoidance of triggering factors (especially stroking, etc.)
   - Oral antihistaminic

Case 141

A 61-year-old male had asymptomatic warty lesions on dorsum of hands and feet for last 30 years. He had similar lesions in his father.

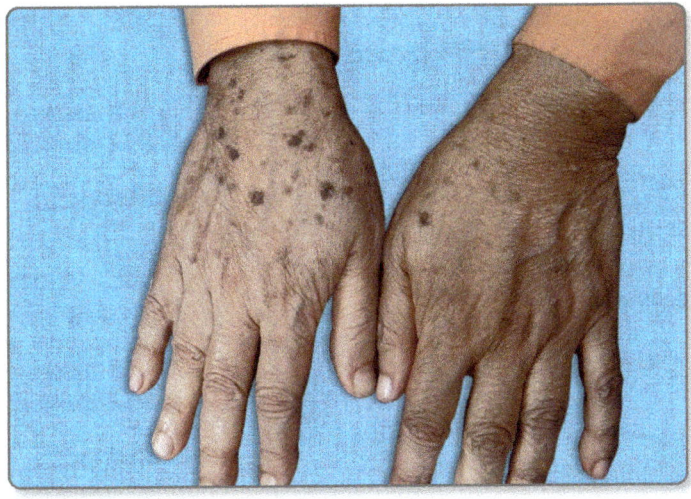

Q. What is the (i) diagnosis and (ii) management?

Answers

i. Acrokeratosis verruciformis of Hopf
ii. Management:
   - Prognosis to be discussed regarding nonmalignant nature and genetic background.

Case 142

A 7-year-old boy had itchy warty lesions on left hand, forearm, and arm since birth which had been slowly increasing as age being advanced.

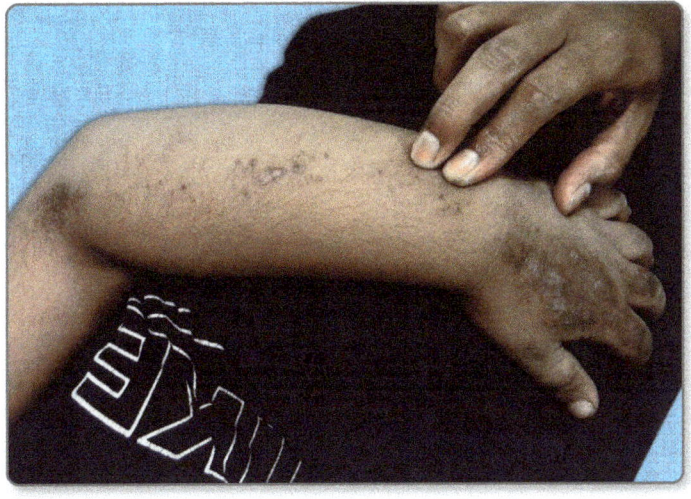

Q. What is the (i) diagnosis and (ii) management?

Answers

i. Linear epidermal nevus
ii. Management:
   - Prognosis to be discussed
   - Electrocautery or cryotherapy may be tried

Case 143

A 72-year-old male had itching and pain with redness on feet in deep winter especially when exposed to cold water.

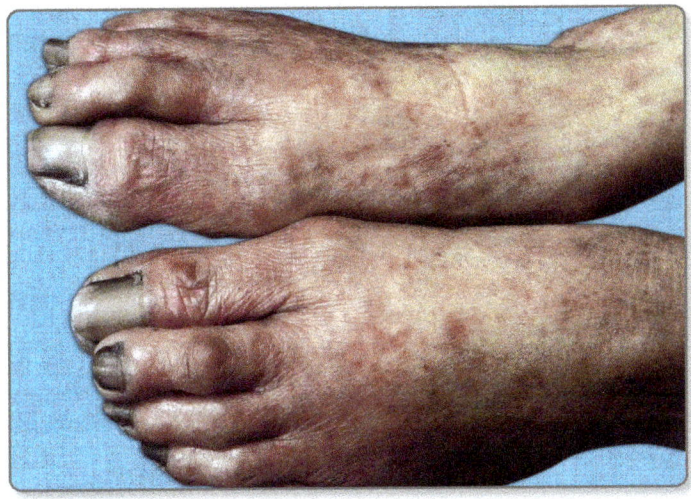

Q. What is the (i) diagnosis and (ii) management?

Answers

i. Chilblain
ii. Management:
   - Avoidance of cold exposure
   - Use of socks
   - Topical steroid

Case 144

A 51-year-old female had acute swelling with pain on corner of right thumb nail for last 1 week. She was a known diabetic.

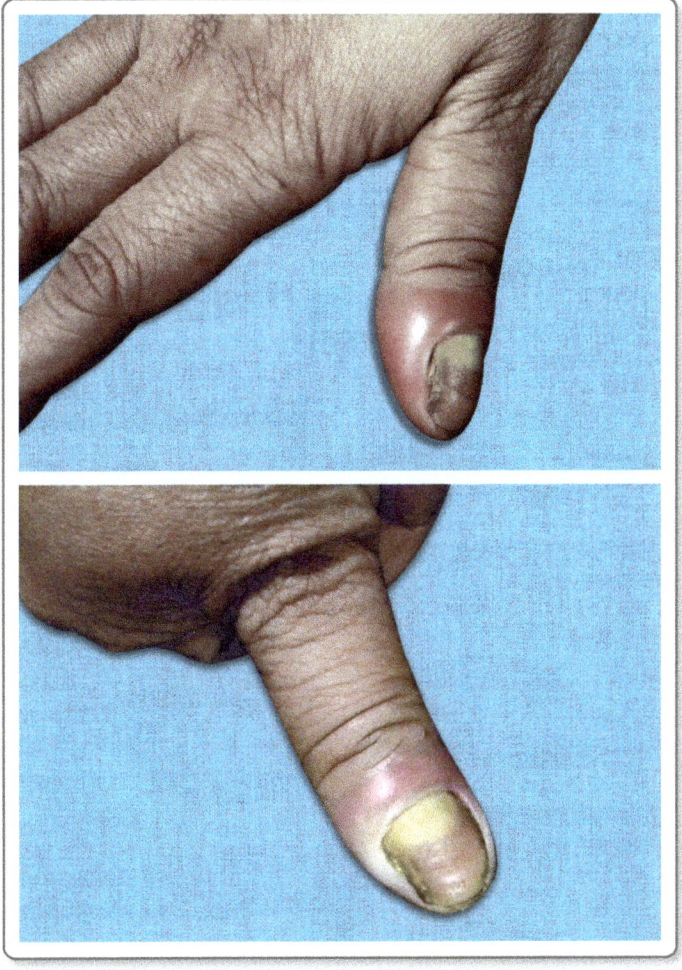

Q. What is the (i) diagnosis and (ii) management?

Answers

i. Acute paronychia
ii. Management:
   - Referral to surgeon
   - Oral or injectable antibiotic
   - Incision and drainage

Case 145

A 34-year-old male had thick warty lesion on side and underneath the nail of right middle finger.

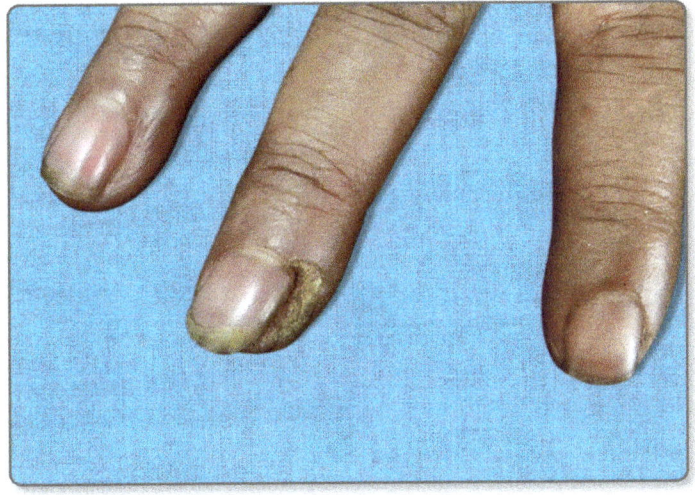

Q. What is the (i) diagnosis and (ii) management?

Answers

i. Periungual verruca (wart)
ii. Management:
   - Chemical cautery
     Or
     Electrocautery
     Or
     Cryotherapy

Case 146

A 68-year-old male had itchy papules with scarring on right forearms for last 3 months. He had regular history of bathing in lake water.

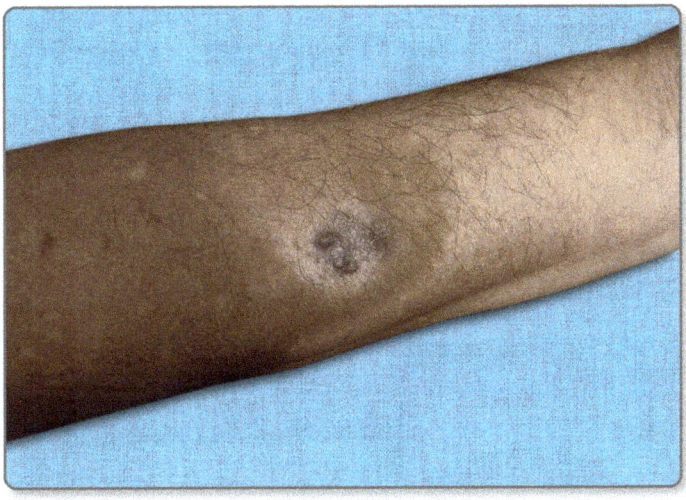

Q. What is the (i) diagnosis and (ii) management?

Answers

i. Swimming pool granuloma (atypical mycobacteria)
ii. Management:
   - Minocycline 100 mg twice daily for 4–6 weeks

Case 147

A 17-year-old female had chronic inflammatory pustules on arms and trunk for last 8 months, which aggravated during humid season. There were no comedones among the lesions.

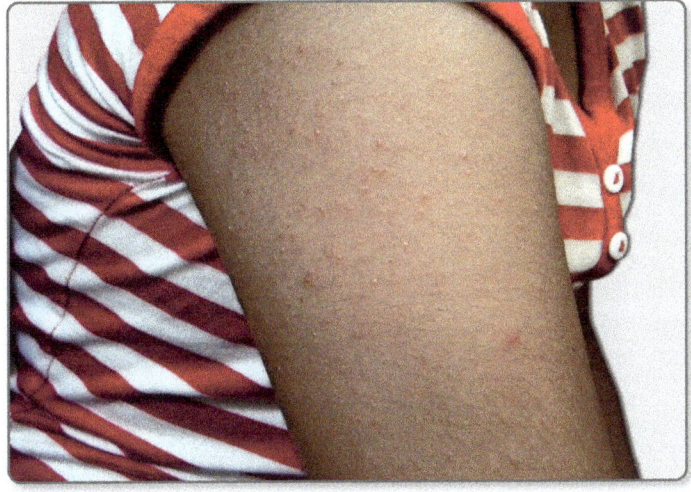

Q. What is the (i) diagnosis and (ii) management?

Answers

i. Pityrosporum folliculitis
ii. Management:
   - Topical antifungal (like miconazole gel)
   - Oral antifungal, if refractory

Case 148

A 45-year-old lady had acute eczematous eruption along hair margin for last 2 weeks. She had history of application of black mehndi on hair during last few months.

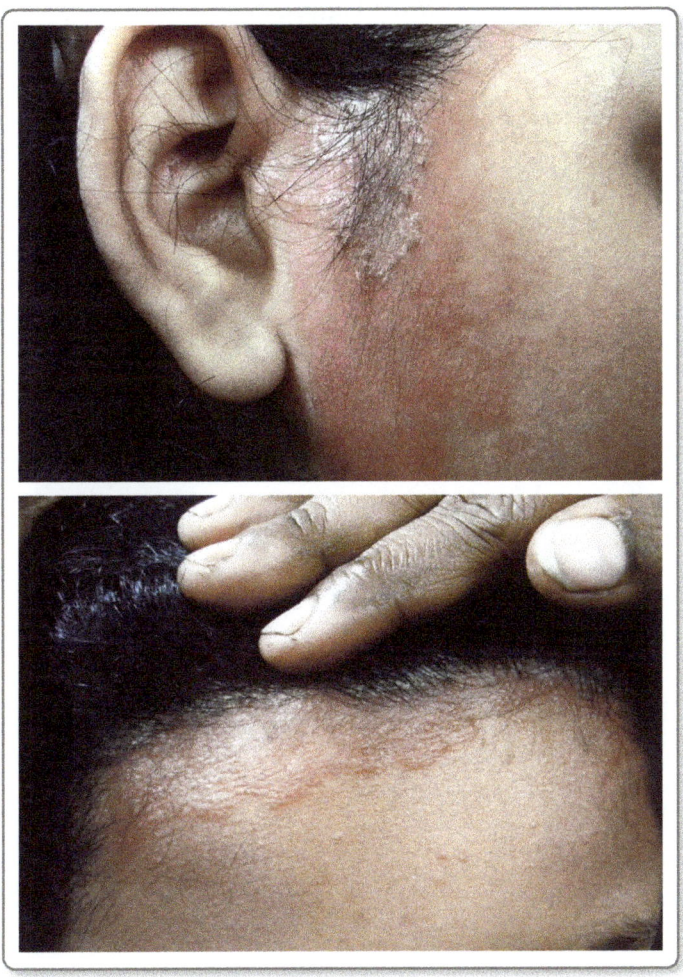

Q. What is the (i) diagnosis and (ii) management?

Answers

i. Allergic contact dermatitis from para-phenylenediamine (PPD) (in hair dye)
ii. Management:
   - Strict avoidance of any PPD-containing dye
   - Topical mometasone lotion
   - Oral antihistamines
   - Patch testing to confirm diagnosis

Case 149

A 9-year-old boy had generalized itching mostly aggravated during night for last 4 weeks. He showed excoriated papules and vesicles at interdigital area and periumbilical area (white arrow) and he has similar episodes in family members.

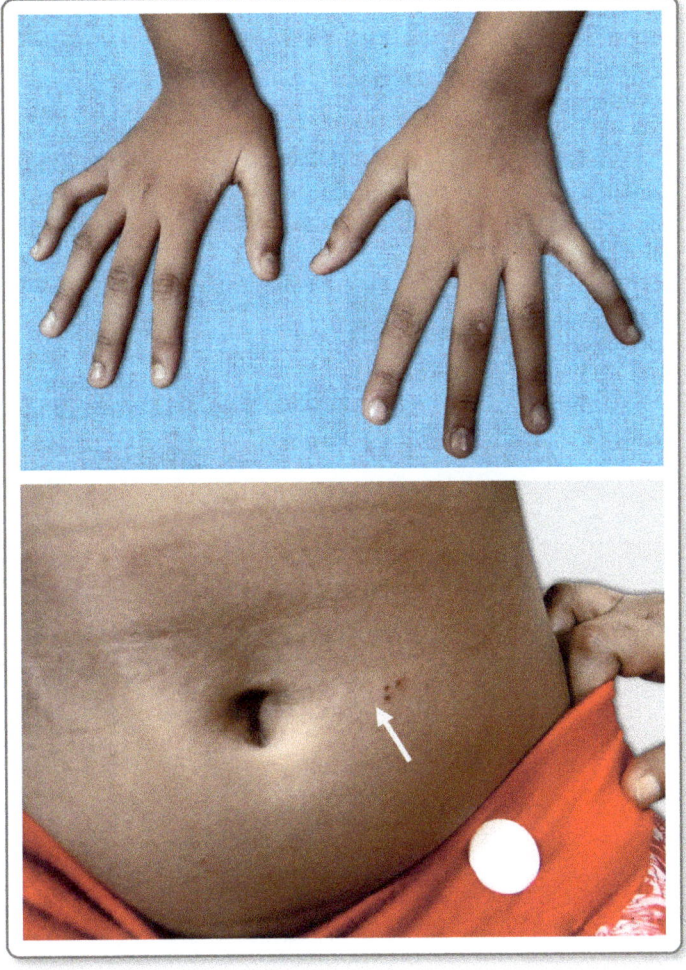

Q. What is the (i) diagnosis and (ii) management?

Answers

i. Scabies
ii. Management:
   - Permethrin 5% cream or ivermectin 1% cream from neck to feet at one night to be repeated next week once.
   - Hot washing of clothes and fomites
   - Oral antihistamines
   - Treatment of family members

Case 150

A 57-year-old male had chronic ulceration on feet for last 1 year. He was a smoker and gave history of pain on lower limbs after walking. His arteria dorsalis pedis was not palpable.

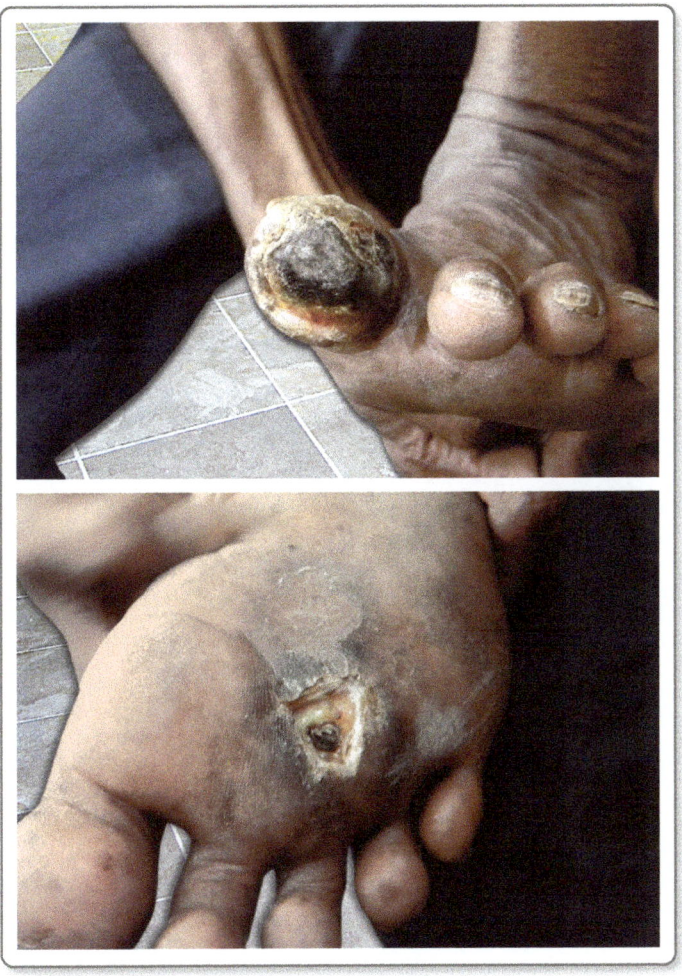

Q. What is the (i) diagnosis and (ii) management?

Answers

i. Buerger's disease
ii. Management:
   - Referral to vascular surgeon
   - Strict avoidance of smoking

Case 151

A 63-year-old male had thick hyperkeratotic scaly lesions on scalp for last 5 years aggravating during winter. The lesions had a well-defined margin along the frontal hairline. His nails showed pitting.

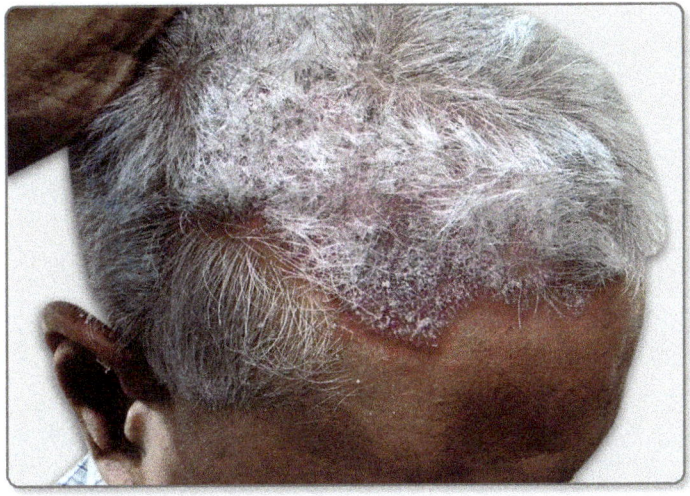

Q. What is the (i) diagnosis and (ii) management?

Answers

i. Psoriasis
ii. Management:
   - Tar shampoo
   - Topical steroid plus salicylic acid 3–6% lotion
   - UVB/PUVA, if refractory

Case 152

A 61-year-old female had been suffering from recurrent blisters on her skin and oral mucosa for last 6 months. She is diabetic and having gliptin group of antidiabetic drug for last 1 year. Her blisters were tense, hemorrhagic, and tend to rupture less easily. The erosion after the rupture did not increase in size. Nikolsky's sign was negative.

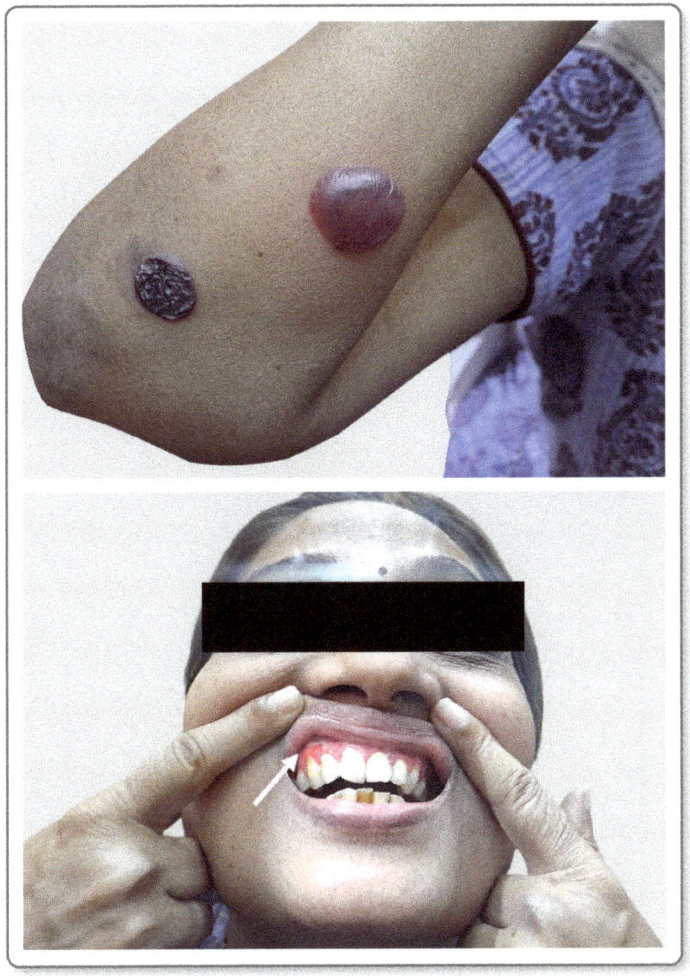

Q. What is the (i) diagnosis, (ii) management?

Answers

i. Bullous pemphigoid
ii. Management:
    - Withdrawal of gliptin group of medication
    - Detailed investigations
    - Oral doxycycline and topical steroid
    - If not responding—oral steroid with mycophenolate mofetil/azathioprine under experienced dermatologist

Case 153

A 19-year-old young adult male had recurrent itchy papulovesicular lesions on limbs and trunk, especially on lower legs for last 2 years.

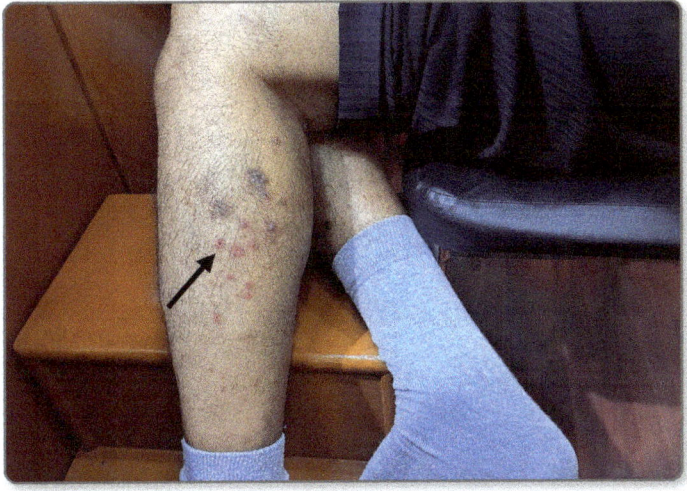

Q. What is the (i) diagnosis and (ii) management?

Answers

i. Prurigo simplex
ii. Management:
   - Avoidance of insect exposure
   - Topical mild to moderate corticosteroids
   - Oral antihistamines

Case 154

A 44-year-old lady had recurrent multiple, painful, irregular boggy, bluish-red ulcerations with undermined edge and purulent necrotic bases for last 2 years. She had associated arthritis as well.

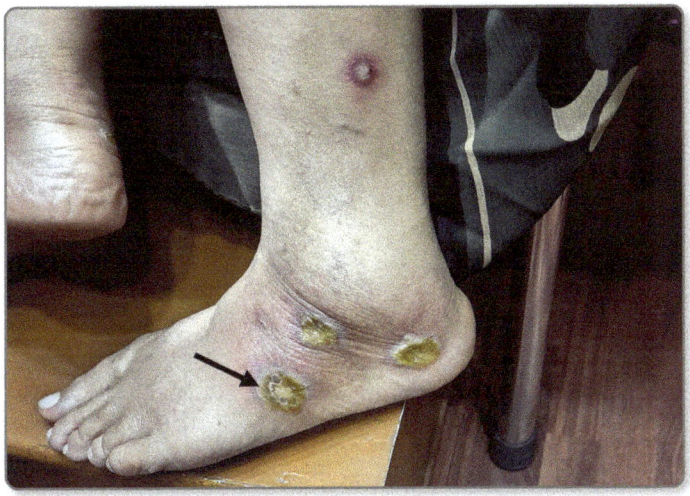

Q. What is the (i) diagnosis and (ii) management?

Answers

i. Pyoderma gangrenosum
ii. Management:
   - Management under expert dermatologist
   - Detail investigations to exclude underlying inflammatory bowel diseases, hematological dyscrasias, and malignancy
   - Referral to respective discipline
   - Ulcer care
   - Oral minocycline, immunosuppressive or systemic corticosteroids or biologics

Case 155

A 56-year-old male had recurrent itchy small papular eruption on forearms, especially after exposure to sunlight for last 1 year. On examination, the lesions had well-demarcated hyperkeratotic border with a characteristic longitudinal furrow, encircling the entire lesion.

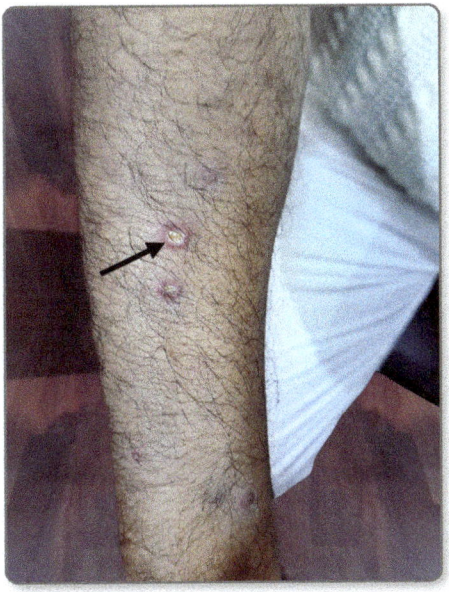

Q. What is the (i) diagnosis and (ii) management?

Answers

i. Superficial actinic porokeratosis
ii. Management:
   - Avoidance of daylight
   - Use of broad-spectrum sunscreen
   - Topical 5-fluorouracil, retinoids or imiquimod
   - Patients should be monitored as these could be precursor for in situ or invasive for squamous cell carcinoma

Case 156

A 42-year-old lady had violaceous (heliotrope) patches with edema around eyelids with flat-topped violaceous papules over the knuckles (Gottron's papules). She had associated polymyositis as well.

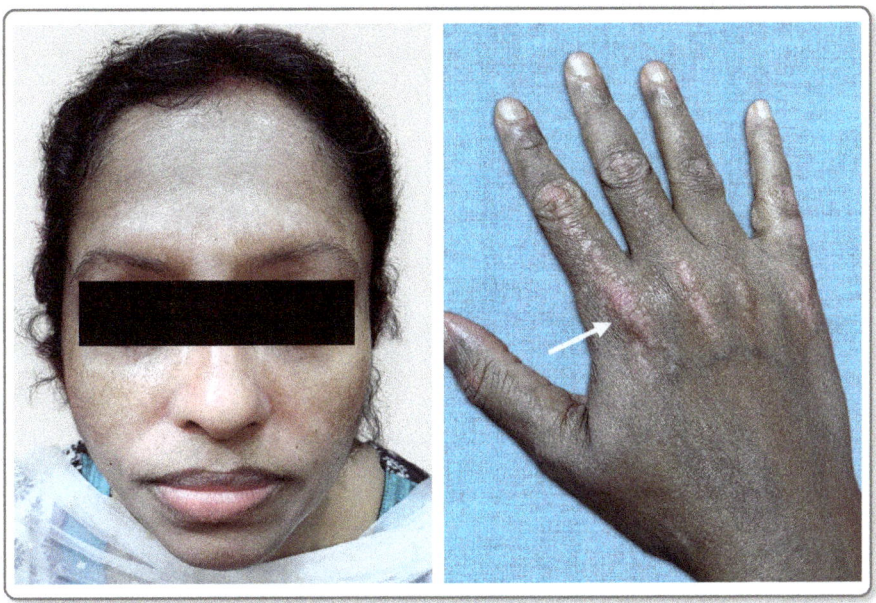

Q. What is the (i) diagnosis and (ii) management?

Answers

i. Dermatomyositis
ii. Management:
   - Referral to rheumatologist and dermatologist
   - Detail investigations
   - Strict monitoring of systemic complications
   - Oral prednisolone
   - Systemic immunosuppressive

Case 157

A 47-year-old lady had recurrent painful grouped vesicular lesions on lips lasting about a week for last 4 years.

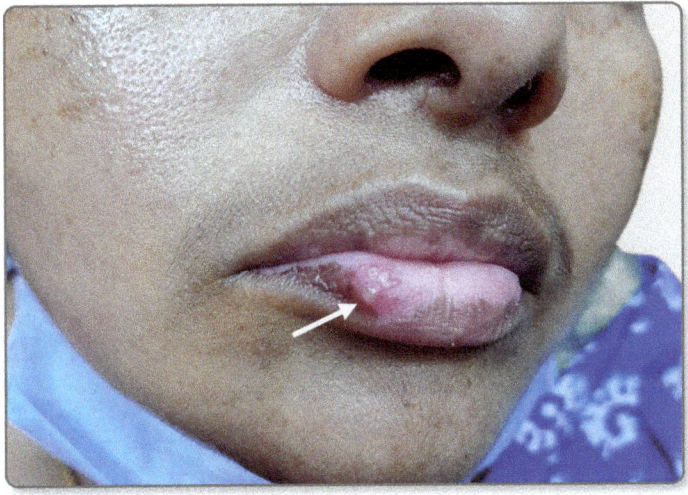

Q. What is the (i) diagnosis and (ii) management?

Answers

i. Herpes labialis
ii. Management:
    - Reassurance
    - Topical 5% acyclovir ointment
    - In recurrent cases, oral acyclovir 400 mg thrice daily or valacyclovir 1 g twice daily for 1 week

Case 158

A 58-year-old lady had palpable (raised) purpura type of lesions along with small necrotic ulceration on lower legs for last 3 months. She had history of chronic dental infections for last 6 months. Her C-reactive protein (CRP) and WBC count were high.

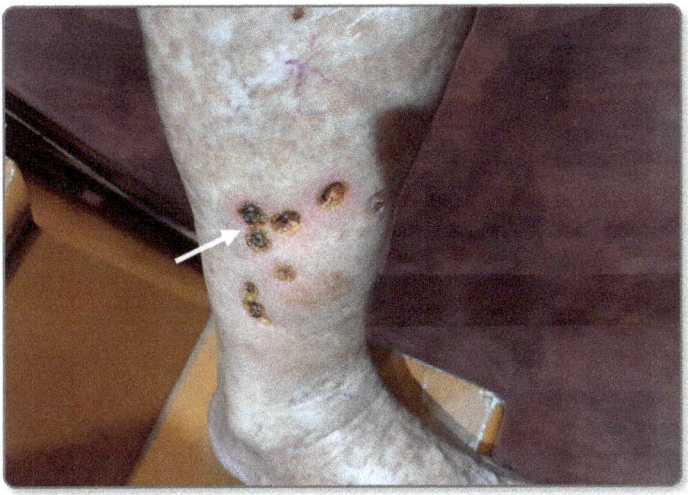

Q. What is the (i) diagnosis and (ii) management?

Answers

i. Hypersensitivity vasculitis due to bacterial infection
ii. Management:
   - Detail investigations
   - To rule out renal and other systemic involvement
   - Referral to rheumatologist if systemic involvement
   - Ulcer care
   - Oral antibiotics
   - Dental treatment

Case 159

A 38-year-old man, manual labor by profession, had these nonitchy hyperkeratotic plaques on the right palm for last 1 year. No other skin lesions were present in anywhere parts of the body and there no associated nail changes.

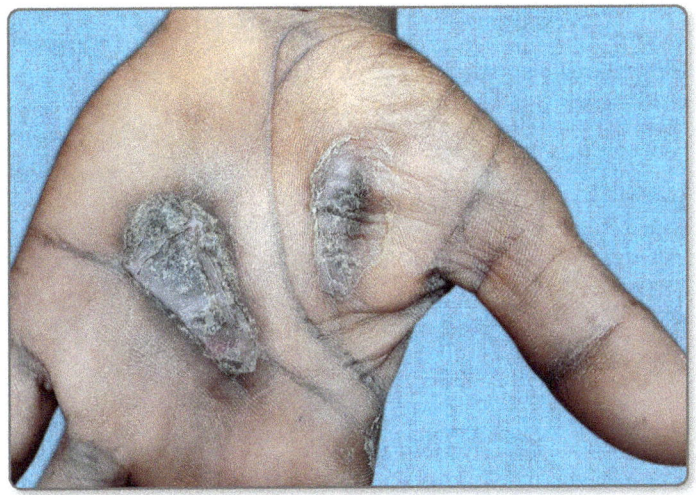

Q. What is the (i) diagnosis and (ii) management?

Answers

i. Occupational hyperkeratotic eczema
ii. Management:
   - Use of gloves
   - Topical potent corticosteroids plus salicylic acid 3.5% ointment for 3 weeks

Case 160

An 18-year-old young girl had irritation, dryness, exfoliation, and cracks on her lips for last 2 years. She had history of mental stress for last 3 years and habit of frequent lip-licking.

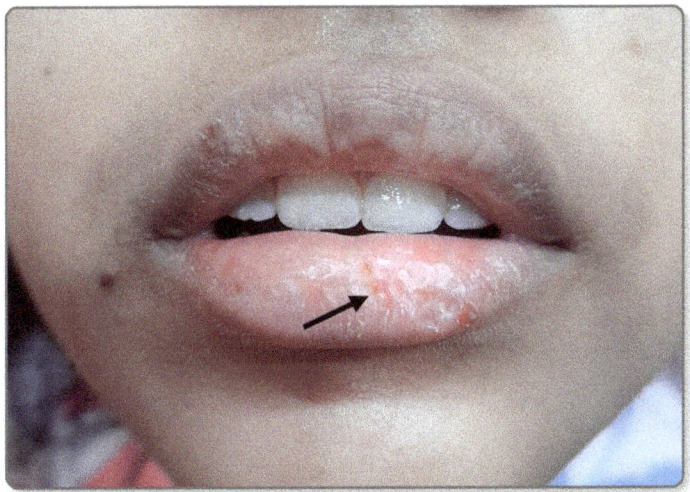

Q. What is the (i) diagnosis and (ii) management?

Answers

i. Factitious cheilitis
ii. Management:
    - Frequent use of lip balm (nonperfumed)
    - Topical mometasone ointment for brief period
    - Topical tacrolimus 0.03% ointment for maintenance
    - Psychological counseling for stress and lip-licking

Case 161

A 57-year-old lady had regular itchy eruption on both legs and feet, which were coin-shaped plaques composed of grouped small papules and vesicles on erythematous base.

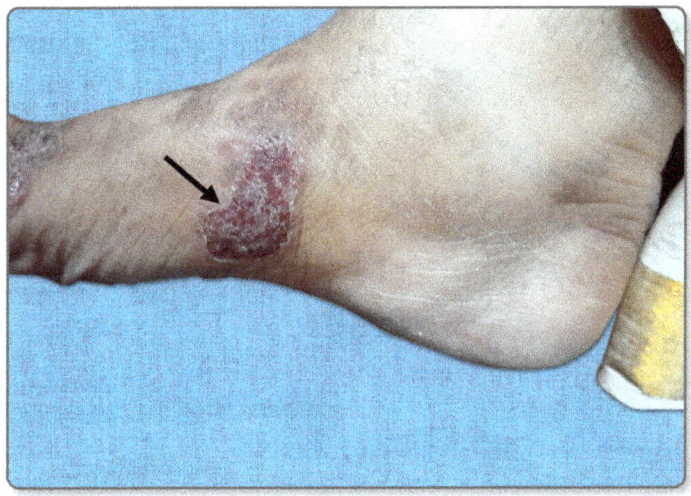

Q. What is the (i) diagnosis and (ii) management?

Answers

i. Nummular eczema
ii. Management:
   - Frequent use of moisturizer
   - Topical corticosteroids
   - Oral antibiotics if secondary infection
   - Oral antihistamines

Case 162

A 41-year-old male had whitish lace-patterned asymptomatic plaques on glans penis for last 6 months. By smear examination, the lesions did not yield any yeast. The person had similar lacy lesions on buccal mucosa for last 1 year.

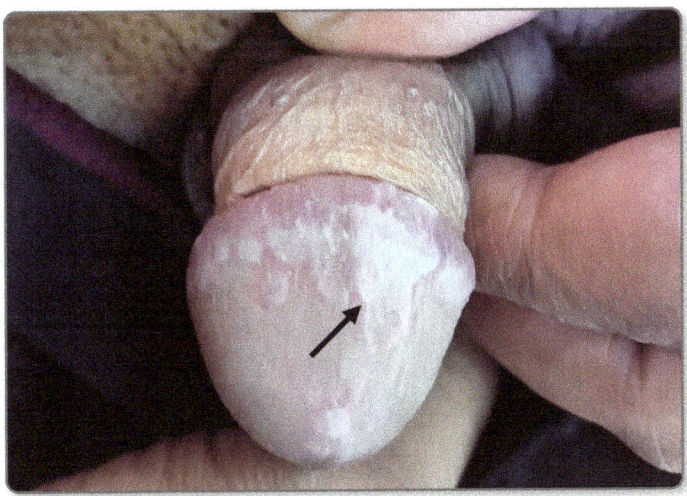

Q. What is the (i) diagnosis and (ii) management?

Answers

i. Lichen planus of glans
ii. Management:
   - Topical low potent corticosteroids for brief period
   - Maintenance with topical tacrolimus 0.03% or 0.1%
   - Management of oral mucosa lesions with topical tacrolimus 0.03% or 0.1%

Case 163

A 59-year-old man had crops of bright red edematous papules and few vesicles, some with central necrosis and hemorrhagic crusting (varioliformis) for last 3 weeks without any fever or malaise on trunk and proximal limbs.

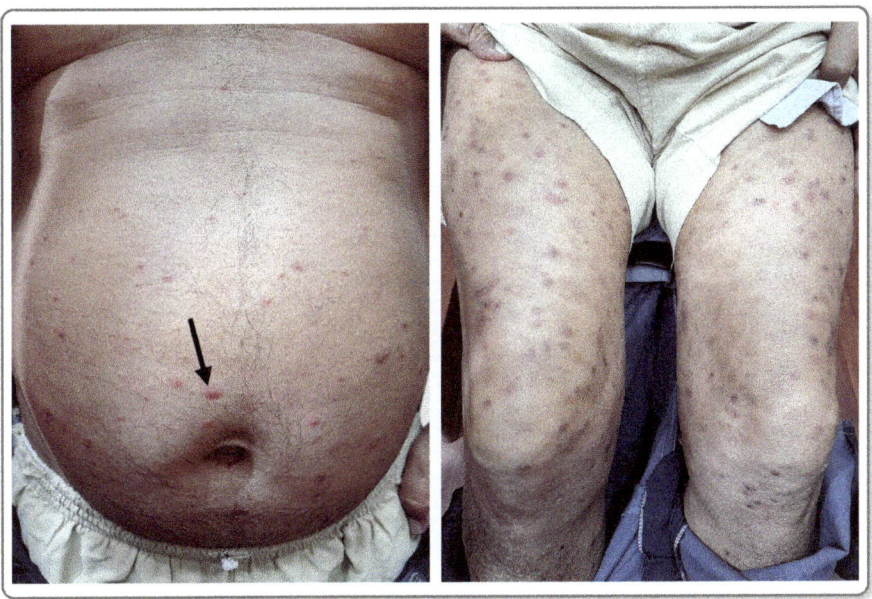

Q. What is the (i) diagnosis and (ii) management?

Answers

i. Pityriasis lichenoides et varioliformis acuta (PLEVA)
ii. Management:
    - Oral erythromycin or tetracycline up to 2 weeks
    - If delayed response, narrow band ultraviolet B (UVB) or psoralen plus UVA (PUVA) therapy

Case 164

A 27-year-old male had atrophic lesions on lower lip with scarring and well-defined border along with ulceration on buccal mucosa for last 2 years.

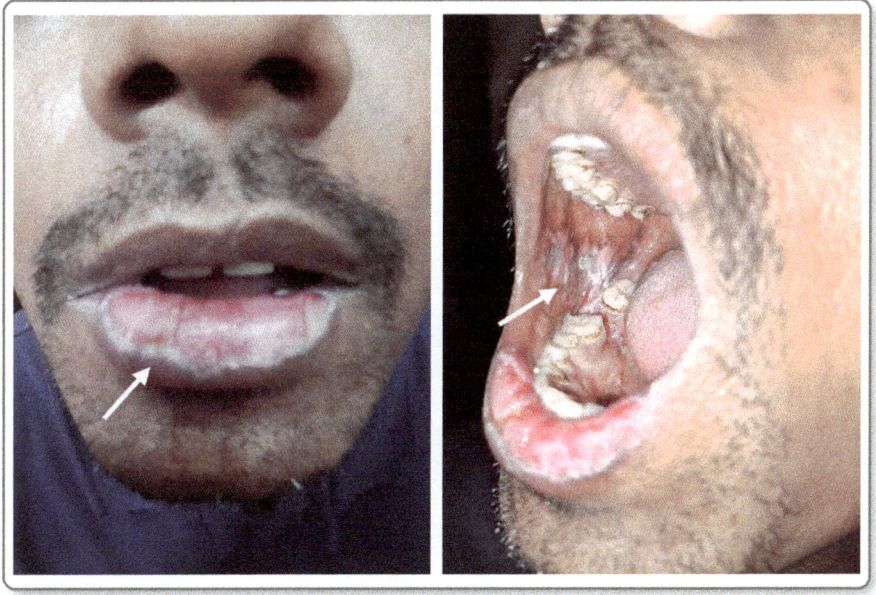

Q. What is the (i) diagnosis and (ii) management?

Answers

i. Discoid lupus erythematosus
ii. Management:
    - Avoidance of daylight
    - To exclude systemic lupus erythematosus
    - Frequent use of lip balm-containing sunscreen
    - Topical low potent corticosteroid locally
    - Followed by topical tacrolimus 0.1% ointment as maintenance
    - Topical tacrolimus 0.03–0.1% ointment on oral erosion
    - Oral hydroxychloroquine 200–400 mg daily by prior and intermittent ophthalmological check

Case 165

A 43-year-old male had depigmented asymptomatic patches on left side of neck for last 3 months. He has been using a new deodorant for about last 6 months.

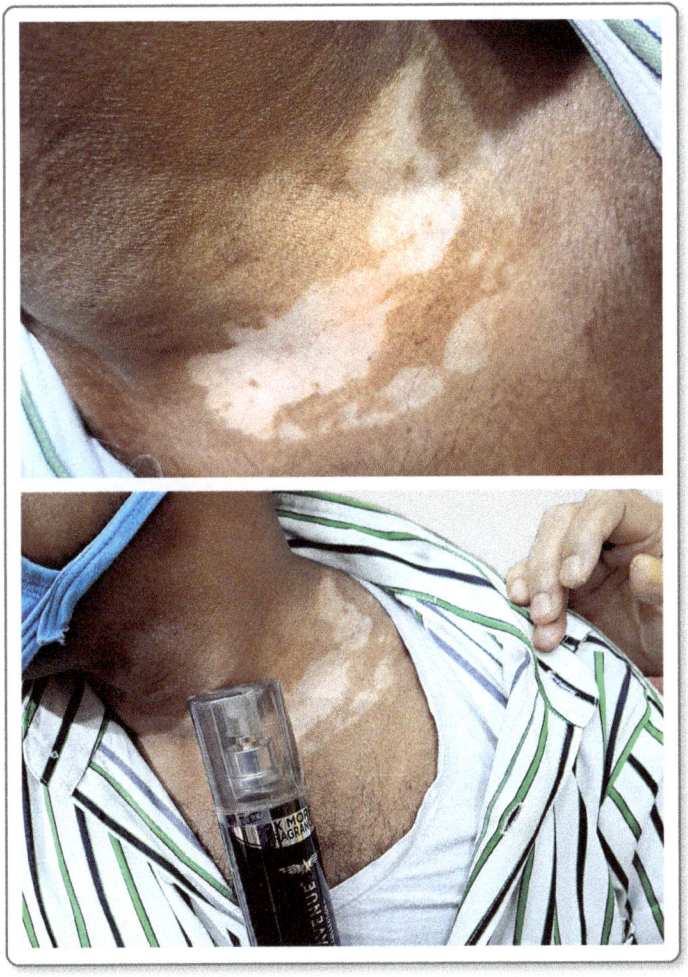

Q. What is the (i) diagnosis and (ii) management?

Answers

i. Chemical vitiligo
ii. Management:
   - Avoidance of deodorants and other chemicals causing chemical vitiligo
   - Topical low potent corticosteroid locally
   - Followed by topical tacrolimus 0.1% ointment as maintenance
   - PUVAsol therapy
   - If delayed response, excimer light

Case 166

A 48-year-old male had itchy, scaly skin rashes on face and external ears without any definite inflammatory border for last 6 months. He had history of applying topical corticosteroid without getting any benefit.

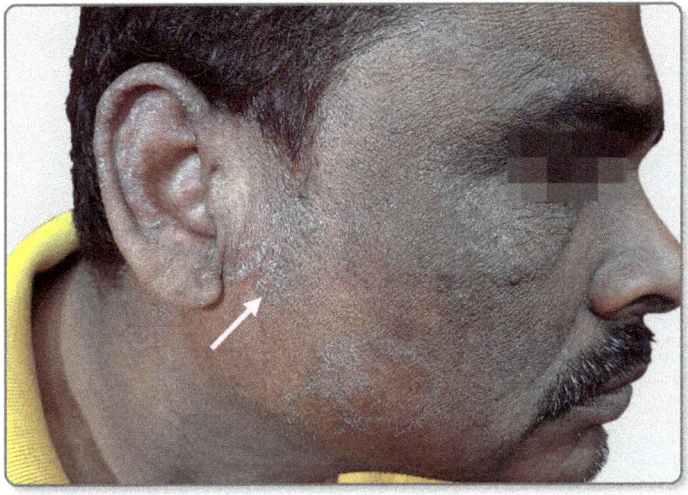

Q. What is the (i) diagnosis and (ii) management?

Answers

i. Tinea incognito or steroid-modified tinea
ii. Management:
   - Avoidance of topical steroid strictly
   - Topical luliconazole or oxiconazole or amorolfine
   - Oral itraconazole 100 mg BD or terbinafine 250 daily for 2 weeks
   - Maintenance of hygiene (avoiding outside shaving, sharing of shaving materials, etc.)

Case 167

A 15-year-old boy had asymptomatic depigmented lesions in segmental area on right side of upper back for last 10 years.

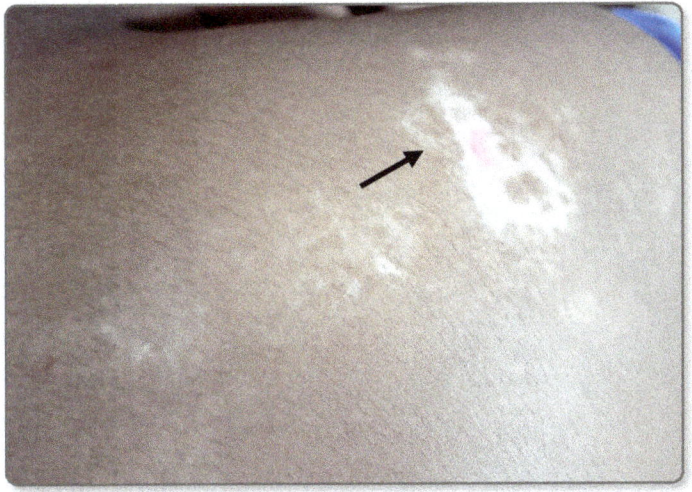

Q. What is the (i) diagnosis and (ii) management?

Answers

i. Segmental vitiligo
ii. Management:
   - Topical corticosteroid
   - Topical tacrolimus or pimecrolimus
   - Topical PUVAsol
   - Excimer light
   - If poor response, Mini Punch grafting

Case 168

A 42-year-old male had an asymptomatic, slowly growing nodule on left side upper back for last 4 years. On examination, the lesion had a central puncta, which expresses cheesy materials occasionally.

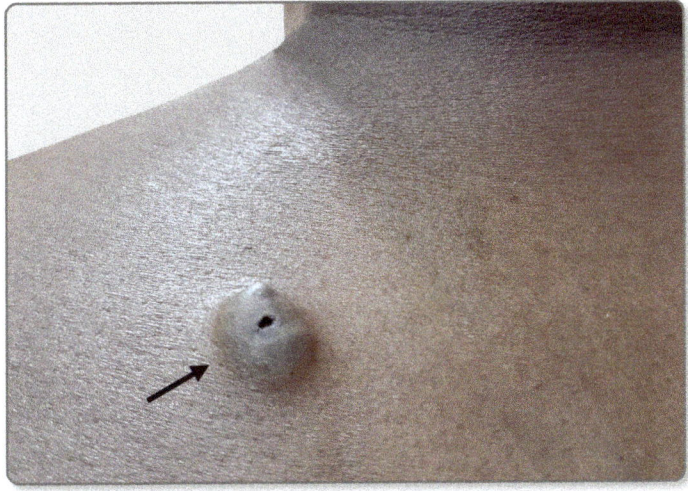

Q. What is the (i) diagnosis and (ii) management?

Answers

i. Sebaceous cyst
ii. Management:
   - Total excision with histopathology

Case 169

A 59-year-old lady had eczematous lesions on both lower legs and dorsum of feet for last 10 years. She had developed sudden swelling, pain, and redness on both lower limbs with high fever for last 3 days after walking through a water-logged road during rainy season.

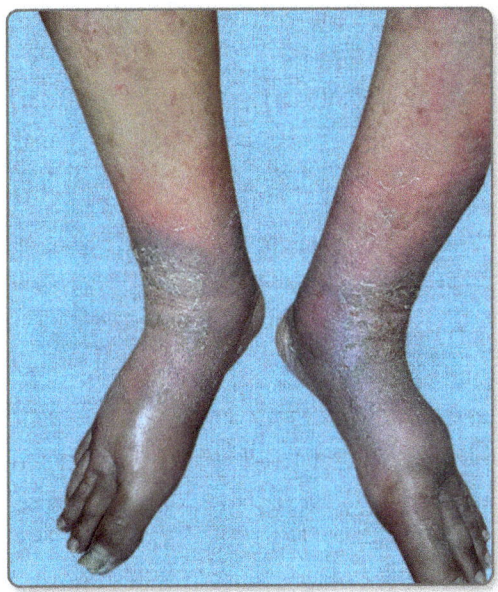

Q. What is the (i) diagnosis and (ii) management?

Answers

i. Chronic eczema with cellulitis
ii. Management:
   - Urgent admission under surgeon and dermatologist
   - Intravenous (IV) antibiotics
   - Leg elevation
   - Strict monitoring for septicemia
   - Withdrawal of topical corticosteroid for eczema, if any
   - Application of bland emollients on eczema
   - Oral antihistamines

Case 170

An 18-year-old male had generalized eruption on whole back, arms, and shoulders for last 1 year. On examination, the lesions had both open and closed comedones.

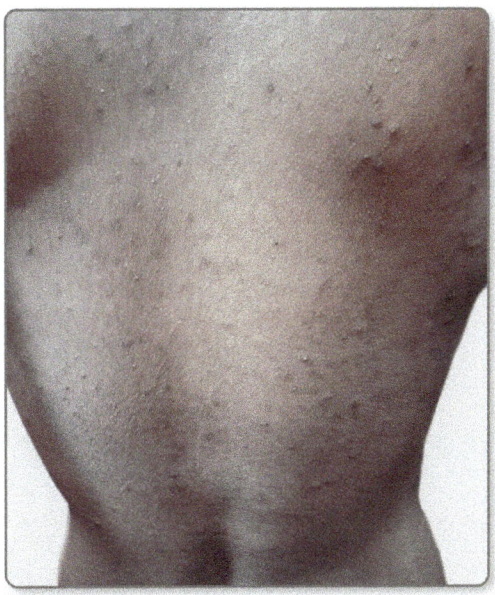

Q. What is the (i) diagnosis and (ii) management?

Answers

i. Truncal acne
ii. Management:
   - Avoidance of oil/oily application and comedogenic products
   - Topical clindamycin gel
   - Benzoyl peroxide wash
   - Oral doxycycline 100 mg OD for 3 weeks or oral lymecycline 408 mg OD for 3 weeks

Case 171

A 69-year-old male has generalized scaly erythematous maculopapular eruption on trunk and limbs for last 2 weeks. He had history of amoxicillin for dental extraction 1 week prior to the onset of these rashes. There were no associated fever, mucosal involvement, or lymphadenopathy. Nikolsky's sign was negative and skin tenderness was not present.

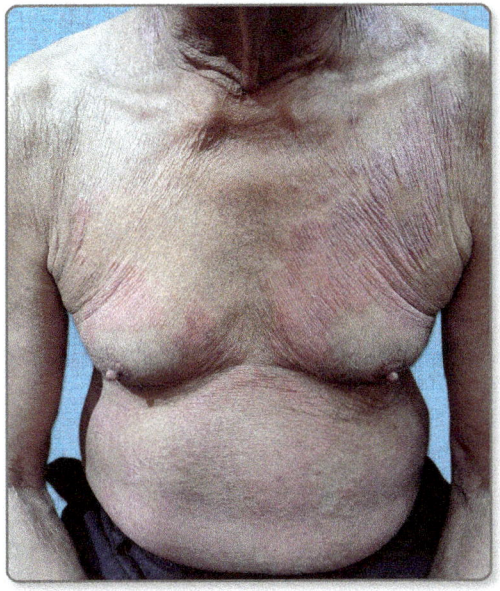

Q. What is the (i) diagnosis and (ii) management?

Answers

i. Adverse cutaneous drug reaction (ACDR)
ii. Management:
   - Strictly avoidance and withdrawal of offending drug and related molecules
   - Topical emollients
   - Low potent topical corticosteroids to be applied locally on specific areas
   - Antihistamines
   - To watch for impending serious adverse drug reaction

Case 172

A 15-year-old girl had excoriated lesions on limbs and trunk sparing the central back for last 4 years. No definite papules or vesicles seen. Her mother admitted that they had marital disharmony for last 5 years.

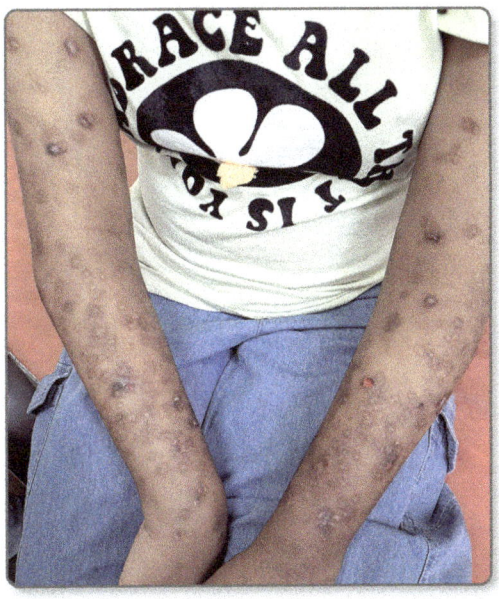

Q. What is the (i) diagnosis and (ii) management?

Answers

i. Neurotic excoriation
ii. Management:
   - Nails to be shortened
   - Calaminol lotion to be applied
   - Phycology counseling and psychiatrist consultation

Case 173

A 19-year-old male had severely itchy generalized eczematous lesions on face, limbs, and trunk since the age of 3 years, which tend to become worse during season change and winter. He had predominant involvement of flexors of limbs.

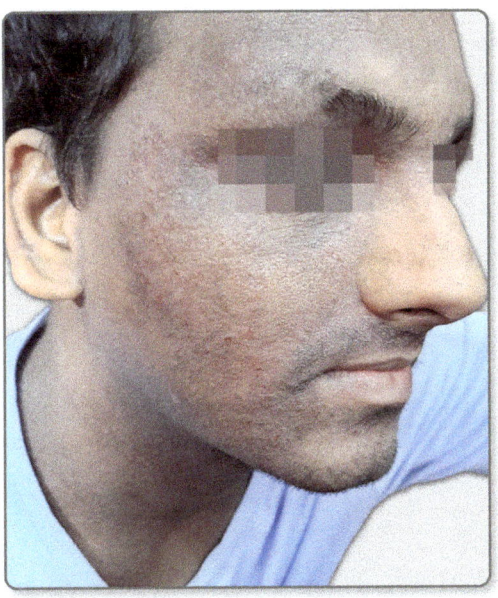

Q. What is the (i) diagnosis and (ii) management?

Answers

i. Atopic dermatitis
ii. Management:
   - *Avoidance of triggers*: Dust, pollens, spray, etc.
   - Topical emollients
   - Low potent topical corticosteroids to be applied locally on specific areas for brief period
   - *For maintenance*: Topical tacrolimus, pimecrolimus, or crisaborole
   - Antihistamines
   - *In acute flare up*: Systemic antibiotics or short course of oral steroids

Case 174

A 24-year-old female had malar flush, photosensitivity, oral ulceration on hard palate, skin eruption on photo-exposed skin along with fever and arthralgia for last 1 year.

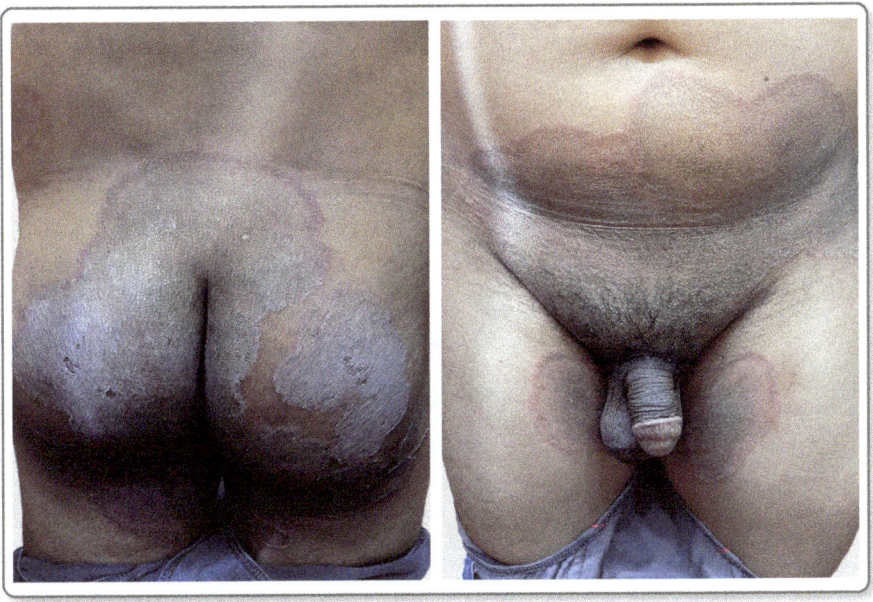

Q. What is the (i) diagnosis and (ii) management?

Answers

i. Chronic and recurrent dermatophytosis
ii. Management:
   - Topical antifungal (luliconazole, oxiconazole, or amorolfin) to be applied one inch beyond the margin
   - Oral itraconazole 100 mg BD or terbinafine 250 mg OD for 4 weeks
   - Antihistamines
   - Maintenance of hygiene (keeping the skin dry, changing of clothes, washing and ironing of clothes, avoiding sharing of clothes, etc.)

Case 175

A 39-year-old lady had severe burning and irritation on back of the neck for last 3 days. She had history application of a pain-relieving balm containing counterirritant there 4 days back for neck pain. On examination, there were erosion, skin peeling, and charred appearance.

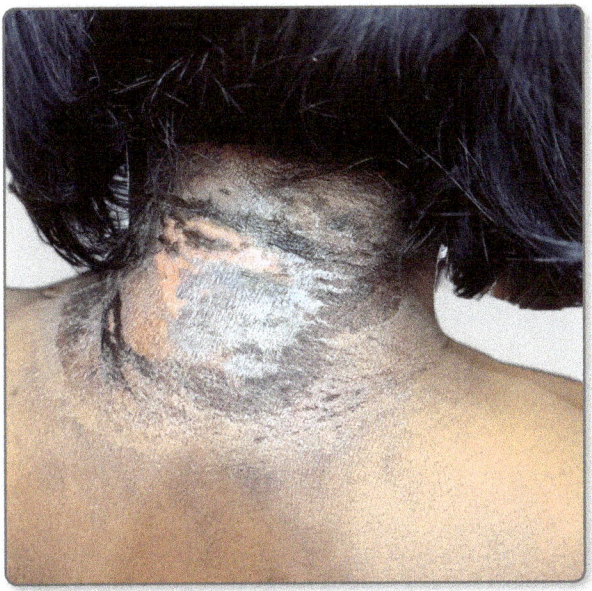

Q. What is the (i) diagnosis and (ii) management?

Answers

i. Irritant contact dermatitis
ii. Management:
   - Avoidance of irritant and also soap, cleansers, etc.
   - Topical mid-potent corticosteroid
   - Oral antibiotic to control secondary infection
   - Antihistamines

Case 176

A 42-year-old man had asymptomatic tiny (1–2 mm) plenty of whitish/yellowish white papules on upper lip for last 10 years.

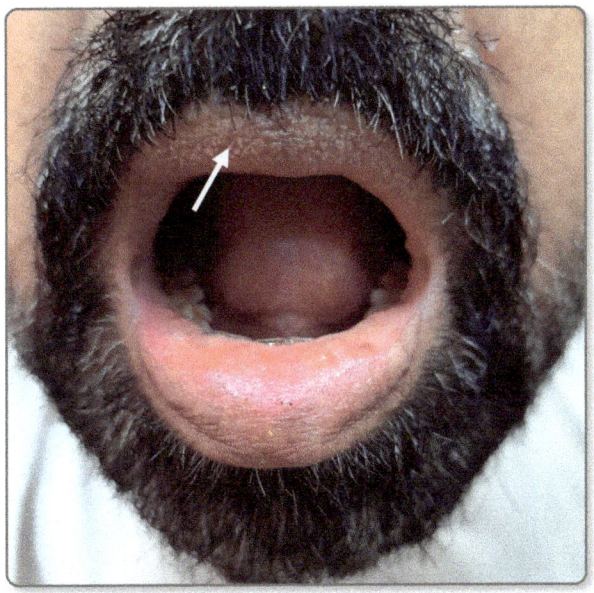

Q. What is the (i) diagnosis and (ii) management?

Answers

i. Fordyce's granules ("Free" sebaceous glands)
ii. Management:
   - No treatment necessary
   - Reassurance

Case 177

A 53-year-old lady had itchy rashes on both hands for last 2 years mostly on interdigital area and web spaces. The lesions were whitish, scaly, and occasionally oozy.

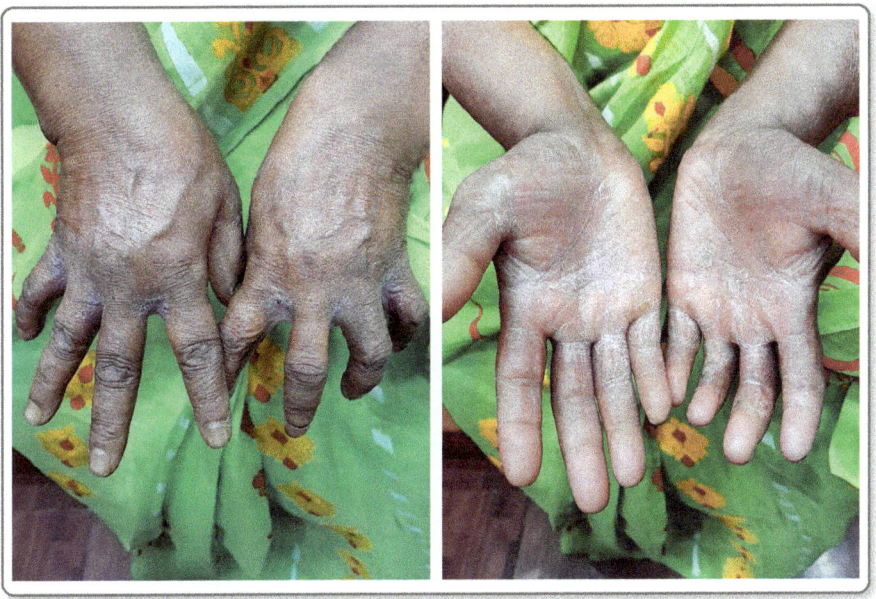

Q. What is the (i) diagnosis and (ii) management?

Answers

i. Candidiasis
ii. Management:
    - Avoidance of water, soap, and detergent as much possible
    - To keep the skin dry after every water works
    - Topical luliconazole, oxiconazole, or sertaconazole
    - Oral itraconazole 100 mg BD for 2 weeks or oral fluconazole 150 mg once/weekly × 4 weeks

Case 178

A 51-year-old lady had rounded erythematous swelling with discharge of sterile pus on right elbow for 6 months following a synovial biopsy operation 9 months back on same joint. The discharge did not contain any bony chips and the patient had no associated fever.

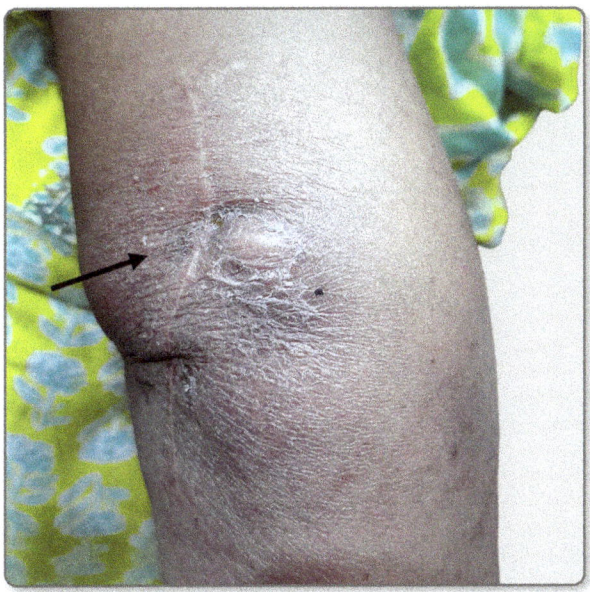

Q. What is the (i) diagnosis and (ii) management?

Answers

i. Postsurgical atypical mycobacterial infection
ii. Management:
    - Oral clarithromycin 500 mg twice daily with ciprofloxacin 500 mg twice daily for 28 days
    - Dressing of the wounds
    - *Prevention*: Proper sterilization and storage of surgical instruments

Case 179

A 17-year-old young male had an asymptomatic dark black sharply demarcated plaque with coarse black terminal hairs on right side of face near right eyebrow and eye since his birth. The lesion has been slowly increasing in size with age.

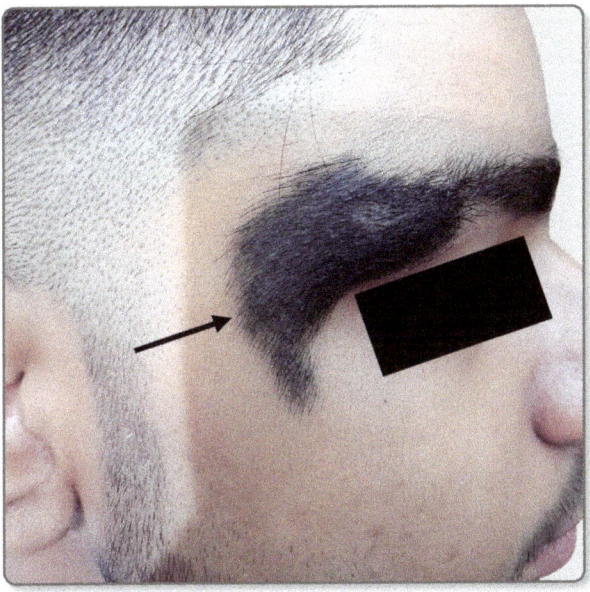

Q. What is the (i) diagnosis and (ii) management?

Answers

i. Congenital melanocytic nevus (CMN)
ii. Management:
   - Surgical excision with full-thickness skin grafting
   - *Prognosis*: Risk of development of malignant melanoma is significant even in the first 3–5 years of age.

Case 180

A 45-year-old female had developed sudden onset pruritic, generalized vesicopustular eruption on erythematous base for last 1 week during hot summer days. She had history of excessive sweating with no associated fever or no prior history of any drug.

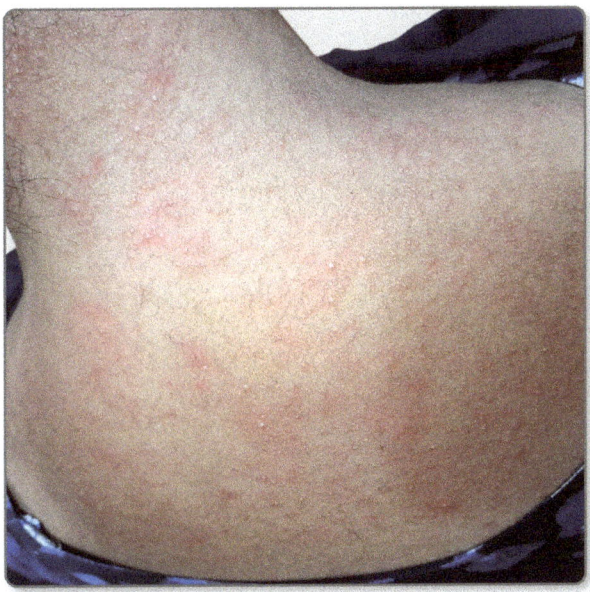

Q. What is the (i) diagnosis and (ii) management?

Answers

i. Miliaria rubra
ii. Management:
   - To stay in cool environment
   - Topical calamine lotion
   - Oral antihistamines
   - Oral antibiotics for *Staphylococcus aureus*, if severe rash

Case 181

A 41-year-old female had multiple asymptomatic warty lesions on right palm for last 8 months.

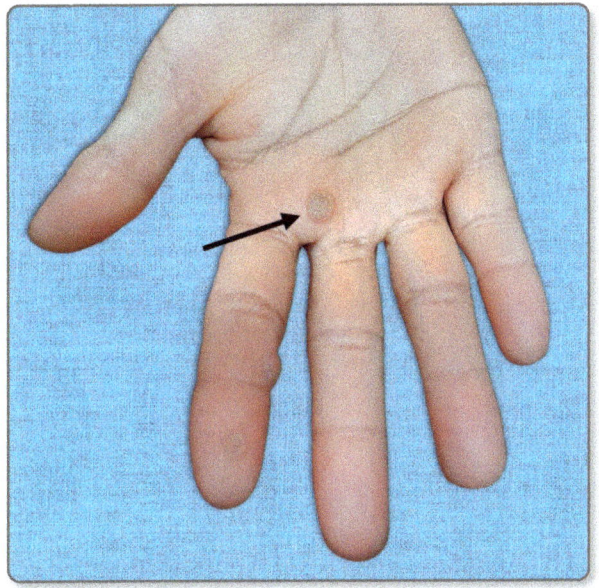

Q. What is the (i) diagnosis and (ii) management?

Answers

i. Verruca vulgaris
ii. Management:
    - Avoid friction and picking
    - Topical tretinoin 0.1% by bud
    - If delayed response TCA cautery by dermatologist
    - If poor response electrocautery or cryotherapy

Case 182

A 61-year-old lady had a slow growing asymptomatic dome-shaped firm nodule on central forehead for last 2 years. On examination, the lesion had a central keratotic plaque.

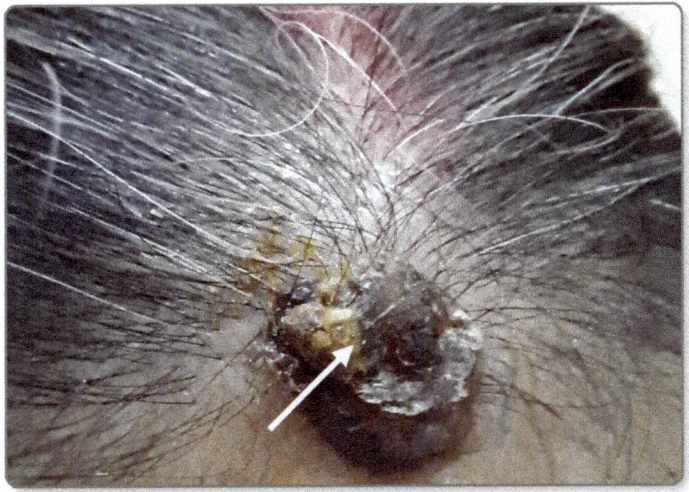

Q. What is the (i) diagnosis and (ii) management?

Answers

i. Keratoacanthoma
ii. Management:
   - Total excision with adequate margin and histopathology
   - *Prognosis*: It is now considered by most as a variant of squamous cell carcinoma.

Case 183

A 48-year-old lady with uncontrolled diabetes had callosity under left great toe for last 2 years which she had paired by lay pedicure process 1 month back, after that she developed nonhealing ulcer for last 3 weeks. She had sensory impairment on the surrounding area.

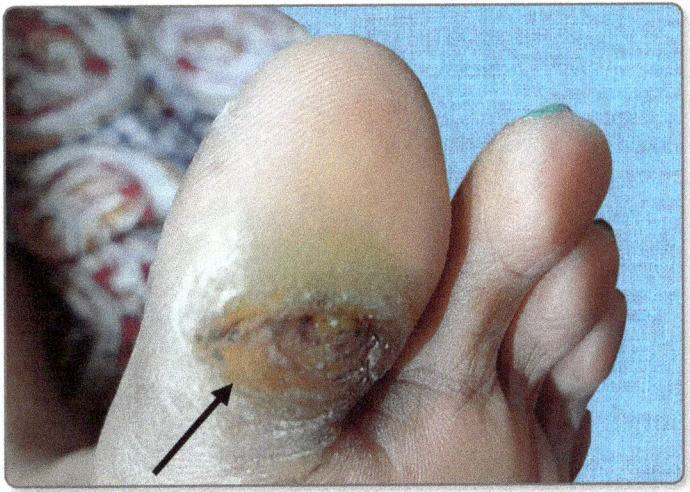

Q. What is the (i) diagnosis and (ii) management?

Answers

i. Diabetic neurotrophic ulcer
ii. Management:
- Immediate referral to surgeon, diabetic podiatrist, and diabetologist

Case 184

A 56-year-old male had a slow growing chronic plaque on right side of face which was sharply marginated, atrophic with scarring and adherent scaling for last 2 years.

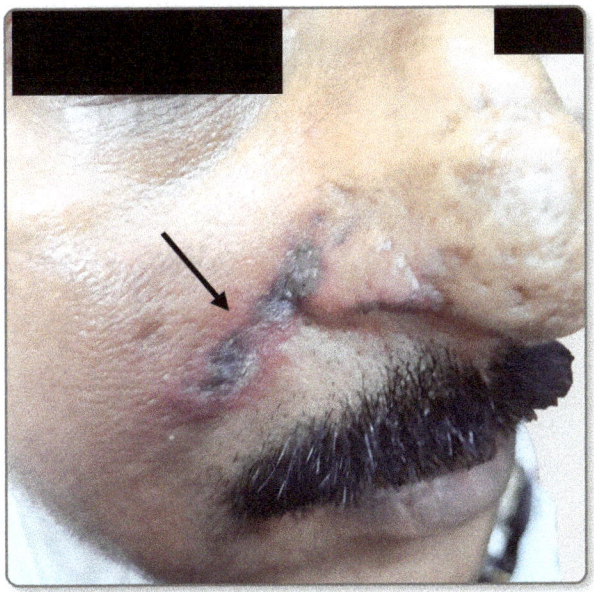

Q. What is the (i) diagnosis and (ii) management?

Answers

i. Chronic discoid lupus erythematosus
ii. Management:
    - Avoidance of UV light
    - Use of broad-spectrum sunscreen with SPF 50+
    - Topical potent corticosteroids for 4 weeks
    - Topical tacrolimus 0.1% for maintenance
    - Oral hydroxychloroquine 200–400 mg daily by prior and intermittent ophthalmological check-up

Case 185

A 16-year-old girl had asymptomatic small papular lesions on arms and forearms for last 3 years. On examination, the lesions were small follicular horny papules.

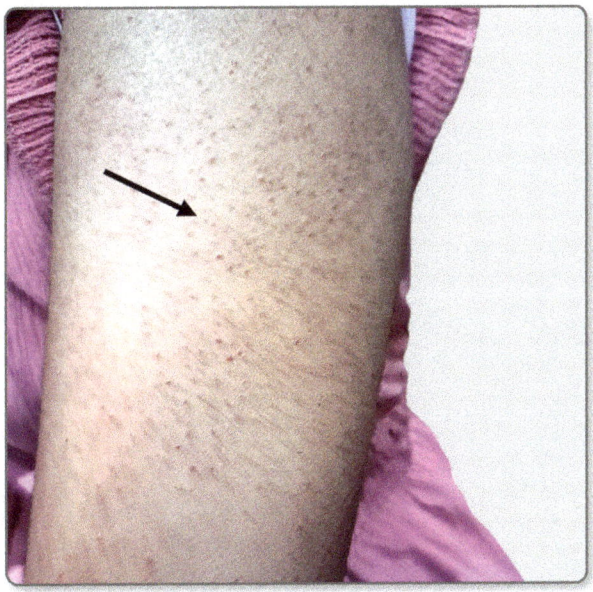

Q. What is the (i) diagnosis and (ii) management?

Answers

i. Keratosis pilaris
ii. Management:
   - Reassurance
   - Topical moisturizer
   - Urea 10% lotion or cream to apply twice daily

Case 186

A 34-year-old male had been suffering from gradually tightened foreskin with whitish plaque on prepuce and narrowing of urine stream for last 2 years.

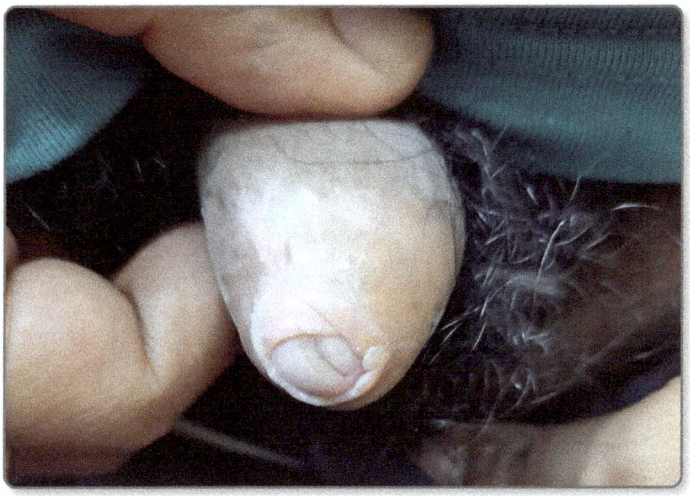

Q. What is the (i) diagnosis and (ii) management?

Answers

i. Balanitis xerotica obliterans or Lichen sclerosus et atrophicus
ii. Management:
    - Referral to urosurgeon
    - Circumcision and biopsy from the glans by urosurgeon
    - Urethral dilatation, if needed

Case 187

A 23-year-old male had recurrent painful ulcers on tongue and buccal mucosa for last 3 years. On examination, the ulcers were sharp, discrete with edematous border.

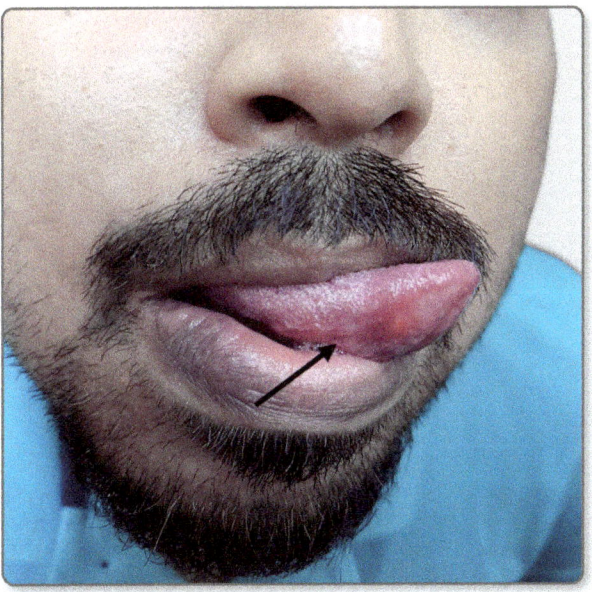

Q. What is the (i) diagnosis and (ii) management?

Answers

i. Aphthous ulceration
ii. Management:
- Viscous lidocaine to apply locally for pain relief
- Topical amlexanox 5% topically 4–5 times daily
- Oral tetracycline or minocycline

Case 188

A 67-year-old diabetic male had sudden-onset painful eruption on right groin for last 1 week. On examination, the lesions were 1–6 mm erythematous follicular-based papules and fragile pustules which tend to rupture to leave yellow crust.

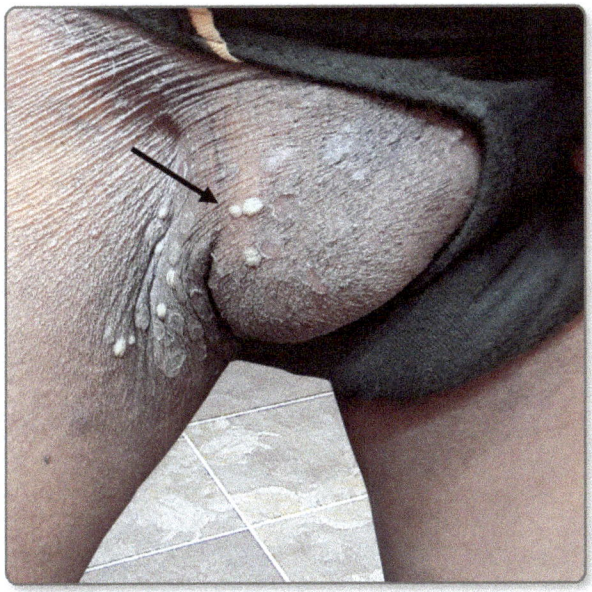

Q. What is the (i) diagnosis and (ii) management?

Answers

i. Bockhart's impetigo
ii. Management:
   - Anti-staphylococcal aureus antibiotic (amoxicillin plus clavulanic acid or linezolid)
   - Topical mupirocin or ozenoxacin

Case 189

An 8-year-old boy had recurrent hypopigmented lesions on both cheeks for last 2 years which were ill-defined patches containing mild scales mostly aggravated after sun exposure.

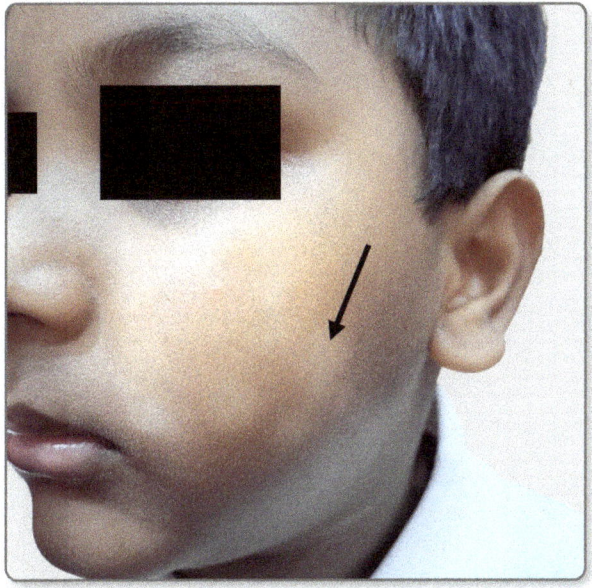

Q. What is the (i) diagnosis and (ii) management?

Answers

i. Pityriasis alba
ii. Management:
   - Physical sunscreen
   - Topical tacrolimus or pimecrolimus

Case 190

A 62-year-old lady had recurrent itchy facial eruption on right side of face aggravated after daylight exposure for last 2 years especially during spring.

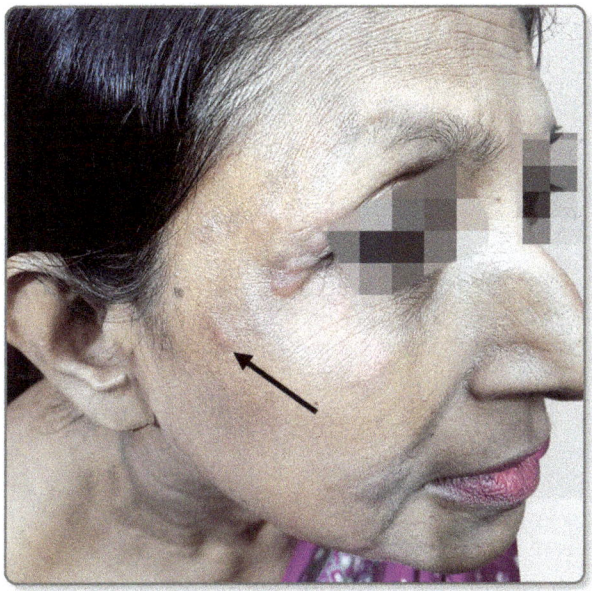

Q. What is the (i) diagnosis and (ii) management?

Answers

i. Polymorphous light eruption
ii. Management:
   - Broad-spectrum sunscreen
   - Topical tacrolimus or pimecrolimus
   - Antihistamines

Case 191

A 22-year-old young female had itchy, erythematous, diffuse hyperkeratotic lesions on palms and soles for 8 months.

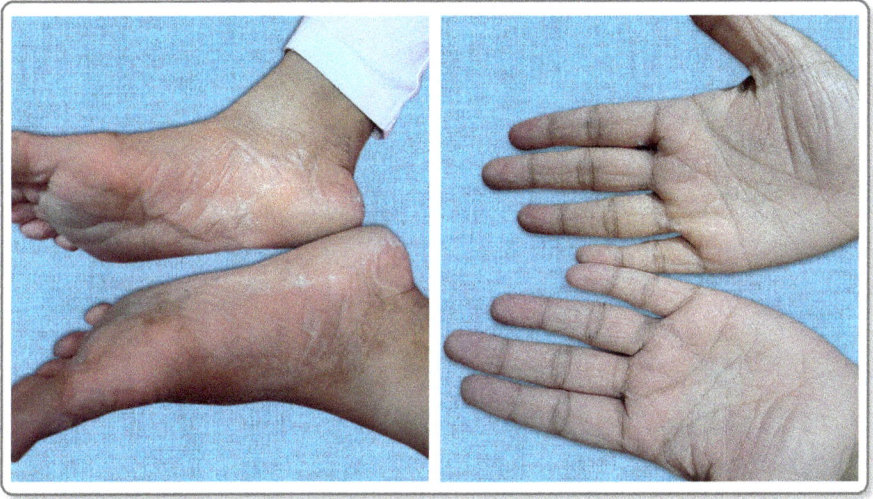

Q. What is the (i) diagnosis and (ii) management?

Answers

i. Pityriasis rubra pilaris
ii. Management:
    - Topical superpotent corticosteroid
    - Antihistamines
    - UVB phototherapy, PUVA or PUVAsol under dermatologist's care

Case 192

A 47-year-old male had pigmented atrophic lacy-patterned lesions on lower lip for last 3 years.

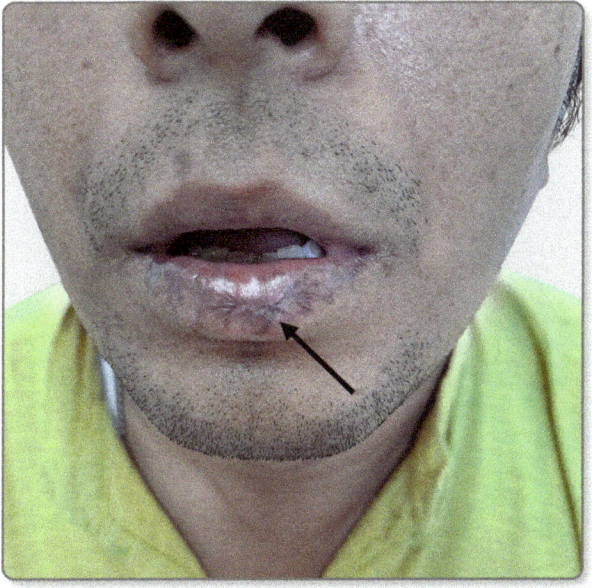

Q. What is the (i) diagnosis and (ii) management?

Answers

i. Lichen planus of lip
ii. Management:
   - Topical corticosteroid for 4 weeks
   - Followed by topical tacrolimus 0.1% ointment as maintenance
   - Lip balm with sunscreen

Case 193

A 21-year-old young man had recurrent painful reddish blister on a particular site of lower lip followed by persisting hyperpigmentation. He gave history of taking ornidazole and ofloxacin combination each time prior to the onset of the episode for diarrhea.

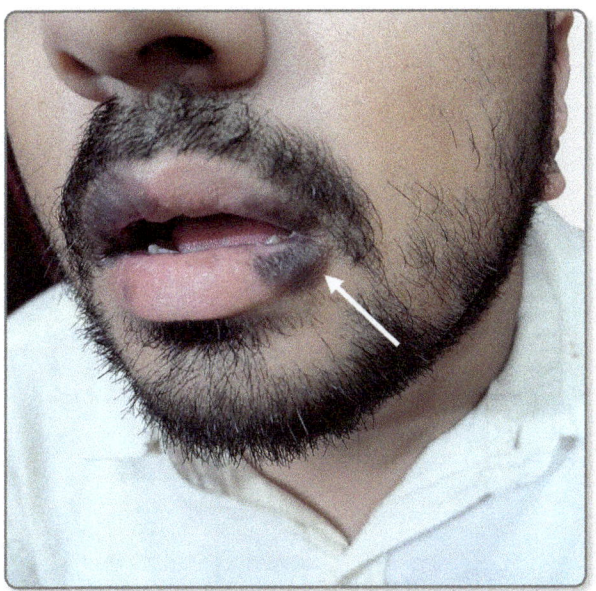

Q. What is the (i) diagnosis and (ii) management?

Answers

i. Fixed drug eruption
ii. Management:
   - Strict avoidance of offending molecules and related drugs
   - Topical corticosteroid for 3 weeks
   - Followed by topical tacrolimus 0.1% ointment as maintenance
   - Lip balm with sunscreen

Case 194

A 68-year-old lady had chronic itchy eczematous eruption on her forehead for last 2 years on her forehead at the site of contact of *bindi*.

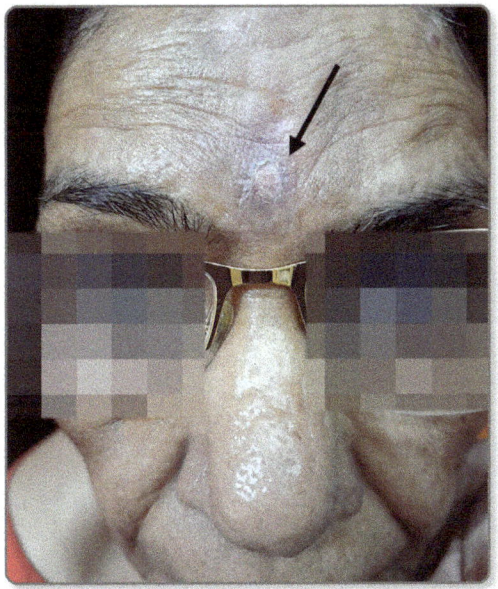

Q. What is the (i) diagnosis and (ii) management?

Answers

i. Allergic contact dermatitis due adhesive of *bindi*
ii. Management:
   - Strict avoidance of adhesive of *bindi*
   - Topical corticosteroid for 2 weeks
   - Followed by topical tacrolimus 0.1% ointment as maintenance

Case 195

A 49-year-old lady had itchy perianal eruption since last 8 months. She had history of application of topical lignocaine-containing ointment for her anal fissure for last 1 year.

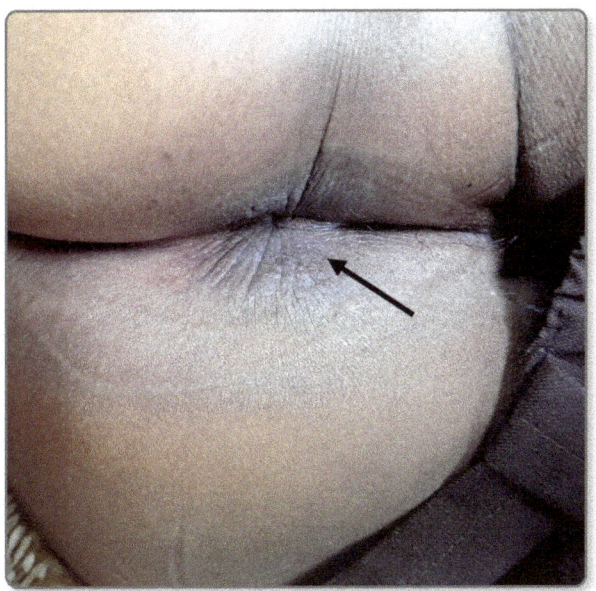

Q. What is the (i) diagnosis and (ii) management?

Answers

i. Allergic contact dermatitis due to topical lignocaine
ii. Management:
   - Strict avoidance of lignocaine-containing cream
   - Topical corticosteroid for 2 weeks
   - Followed by topical tacrolimus 0.1% ointment as maintenance
   - Antihistamines

Case 196

A 76-year-old lady had a chronic slow growing ulcer on her left pinna for last 3 years. On examination, the ulcer had a rolled border.

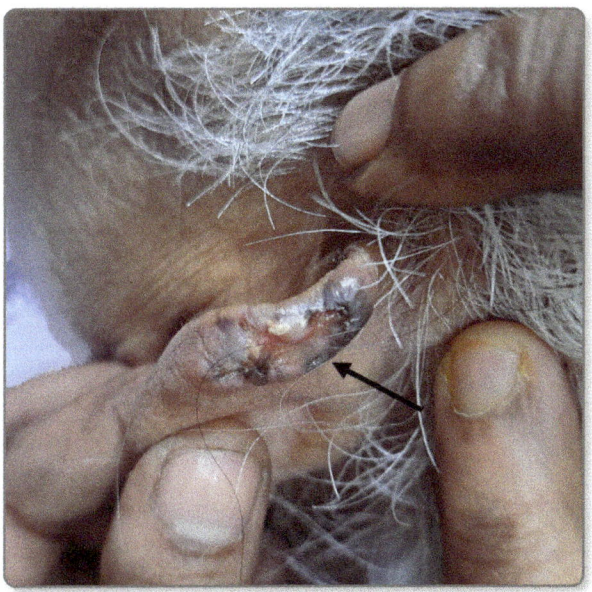

Q. What is the (i) diagnosis and (ii) management?

Answers

i. Basal cell carcinoma
ii. Management:
   - Surgical excision

Case 197

A 49-year-old lady had multiple depressed plaques with "cliff sign" without any induration on limbs and trunk for last 1 year.

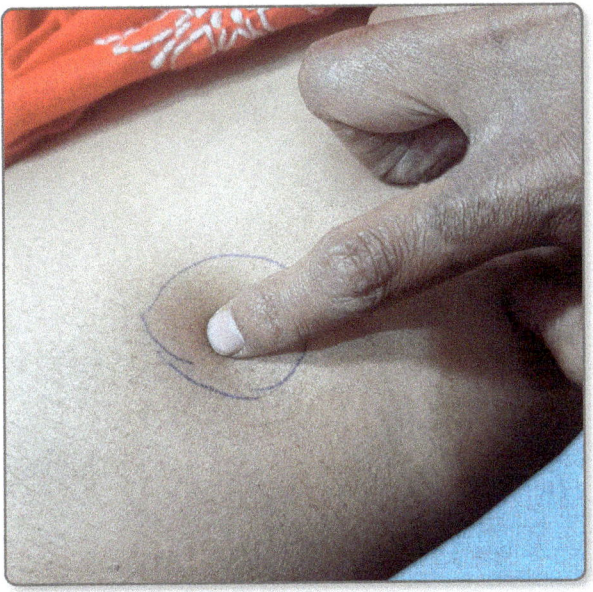

Q. What is the (i) diagnosis and (ii) management?

Answers

i. Atrophoderma of Pasini and Pierini
ii. Management:
   - No definite treatment
   - In patients with positive *Borrelia Burgdorferi* antibody titer oral doxycycline 200 mg/daily for 2–3 weeks

Case 198

A 34-year-old lady had generalized maculopapular brownish–red lesions including few papulosquamous lesions on palms and soles. She had associated fever, malaise, and lymphadenopathy. There were no preceding drug history. Blood VDRL test was positive in dilution of 1:60 and TPHA was positive.

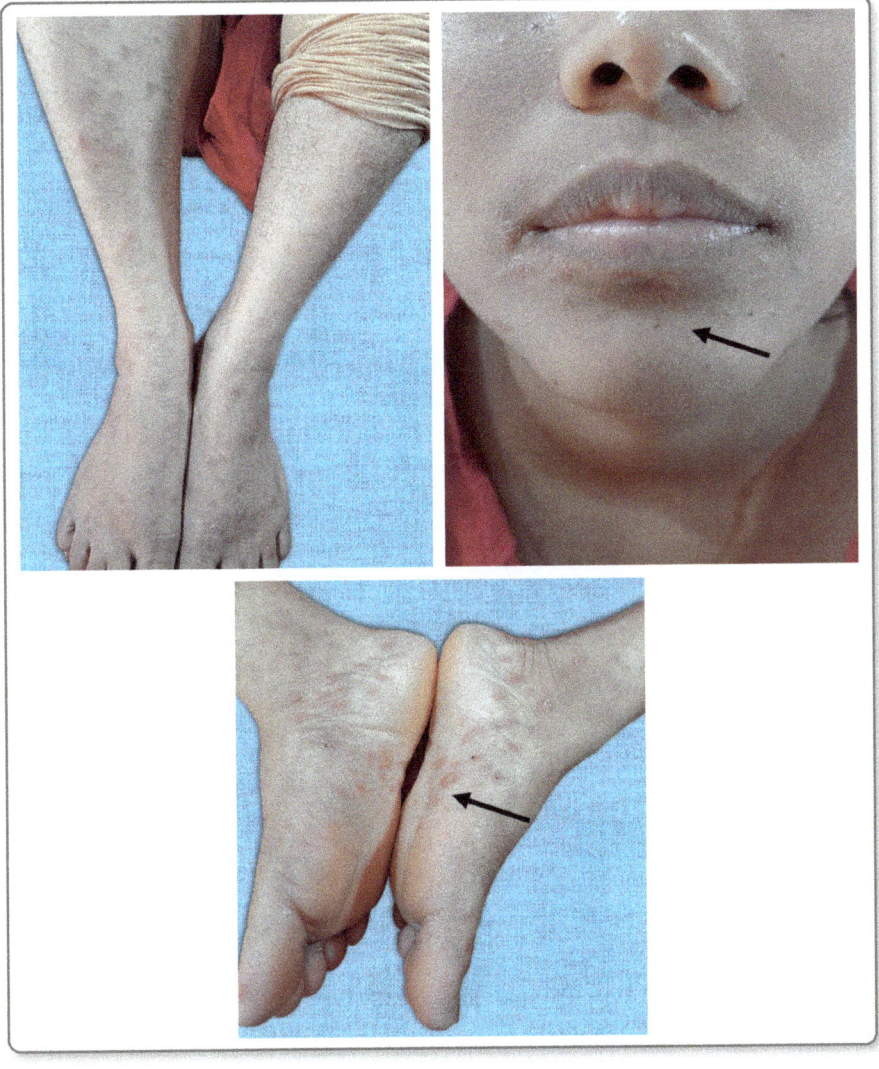

Q. What is the (i) diagnosis and (ii) management?

Answers

i. Secondary syphilis
ii. Management:
   - Intramuscular benzathine penicillin G 2.4 million units in single dose (if allergic to penicillin after desensitization of penicillin)

Case 199

A 69-year-old female had nonhealing ulceration on lateral side of dorsum of right foot for last 6 months which tend to become painful at night. The ulcer was punched out with sharply demarcated border with surrounding erythema.

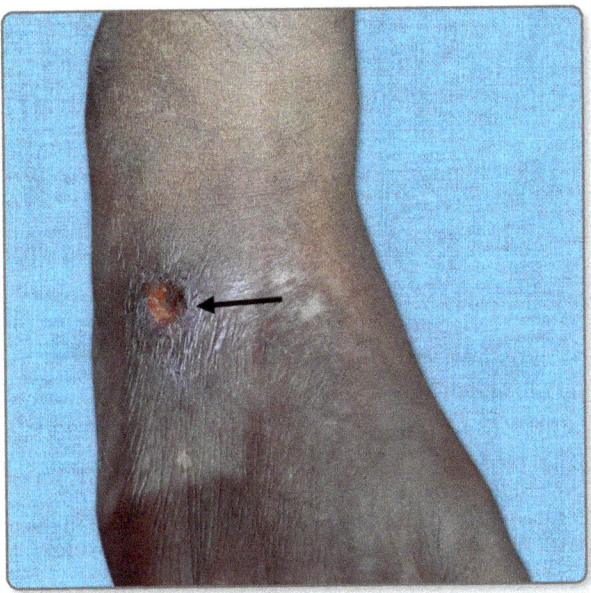

Q. What is the (i) diagnosis and (ii) management?

Answers

i. Chronic leg ulcer (arterial)
ii. Management:
    ➢ Swab from the ulcer for bacterial culture and sensitivity
    ➢ Regular and proper dressing of ulcer
    ➢ Arterial and venous Doppler study of both lower limbs
    ➢ Consultation with vascular surgeon

Case 200

A 68-year-old male had generalized blisters on trunk, limbs, and face for last 6 months with oral erosions. The blisters were flaccid, tend to rupture easily and after rupture area of erosion increased in size as compared to the blister. Nikolsky sign was positive.

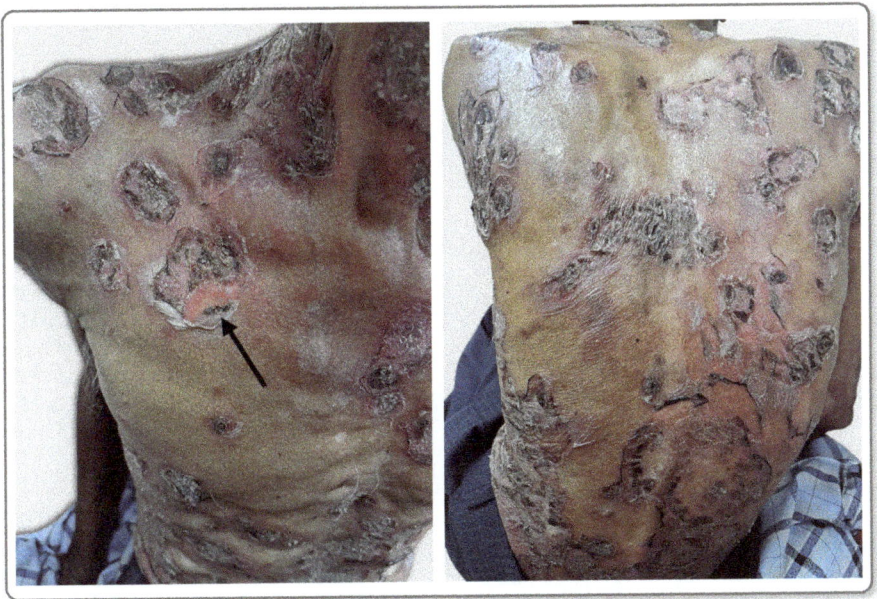

Q. What is the (i) diagnosis and (ii) management?

Answers

i. Pemphigus vulgaris
ii. Management:
- ➤ Urgent admission under dermatologist and physician for investigation and treatment.

Case 201

A 68-year-old male had discrete, sessile, papilloma-like growth on right groin and lower pubic region for last 1 year. He had history of sexual exposure to unknown females. Blood VDRL test and TPHA were negative.

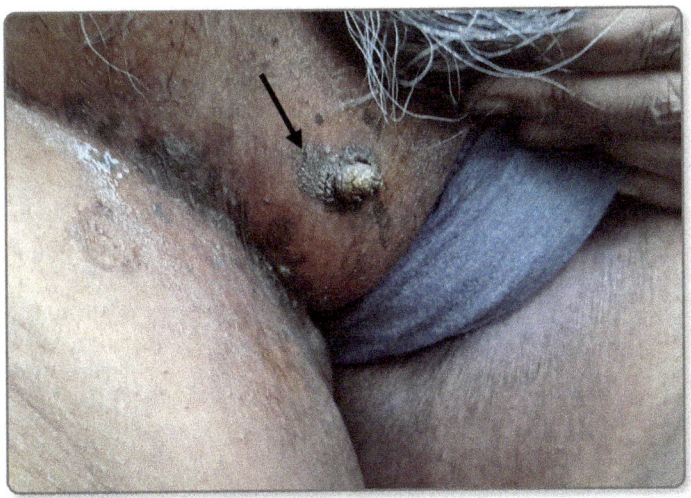

Q. What is the (i) diagnosis and (ii) management?

Answers

i. Condyloma acuminata
ii. Management:
   - Topical podophyllin or imiquimod under dermatologist's supervision
   - Cryotherapy or electrosurgery if refractory

Index

A

Acanthosis nigricans 42, 84
Acitretin 210
Acne 101, 214
　keloidalis 38
nuchae 110
　nodularis 80
　scar management 102
　treatment of 38, 80
　vulgaris 164
Acneiform eruption, painful 109
Acrochordon 272
Actinic porokeratosis, superficial 310
Actinomycetoma 248
Acyclovir 120, 314
Adaferin 102
Adapalene 164
Adrenal tumor 154
Allergens, causative 204
Allergic patch test 36, 142, 202, 204
Allergic purpura 54
Allergy, insect 126
Allopurinol 266
　immediate withdrawal of 266
Alopecia
　androgenetic 154
　areata 174
Aluminum chloride hexahydrate 114
Amalgam 98
Amlexanox 374
Amorolfine 18, 46, 128, 152, 348
Amoxicillin 106, 211
　plus clavulanic acid 376
Anesthetic limbs, care of 12
Angioedema, acquired 264
Angiokeratoma scroti 90
Angiotensin-converting enzyme
　　inhibitor 263
Angiotensin-receptor blocking agents 264
Antibiotics
　short course of 136
　systemic 262
Anti-bradykinin agent 264
Antidiabetic 226

Antifungal 190, 294
　treatment, systemic 47
Antihistamines 36, 98, 126, 136, 186,
　194, 212, 268, 296, 250, 350, 382
Antinuclear antibody test 32
Anti-staphylococcal aureus antibiotic
　376
Aphthous ulceration 374
Apremilast 44, 210
Arsenic keratosis 254
Arteria dorsalis pedis 299
Arthralgia 191
Arthritis, psoriatic 44
Asthma 241
Atopic dermatitis 160, 242, 278, 346
　specific treatment of 160
Atopic triggers, avoidance of 242
Atrophy 165
Auspitz sign 215
Axillae 106, 271
Azathioprine 226, 304
Azelaic acid 68

B

Balanitis xerotica obliterans 150, 372
Basal cell carcinoma 392
Bazin erythema induratum 100
Behçet's disease 94
Benzathine penicillin 396
Benzoyl peroxide 38, 68, 82, 102, 110,
　164, 168, 236, 340
Bernhardt's syndrome 122
Beta-hemolytic *streptococcus* 88
Bexarotene, topical 124
Bindi, adhesive of 388
Black mehndi, history of application of
　295
Bland emollients 338
Blisters, recurrent 303
Blood sugar profile 42
Bockhart's impetigo 376
Body surface area 206
Borderline tuberculoid 232
Borrelia burgdorferi antibody titer 394

Bronchial spasm 241
Buccal mucosa 9
Buerger's disease 300
Bullous pemphigoid 226, 304

C

Café au lait macules 129
Calamine 54, 244
Calaminol 344
Calcipotriol 60
Calcium channel blockers 200
Candida overgrowth 10
Candidiasis 354
Ceftriaxone 230
Cellulitis 338
Cement dust 194
Cephalexin 88
Chancroid 230
Chemical cautery 72, 260, 290
Chemotherapy, systemic 124
Chickenpox 22
Chilblain 286
Chlorhexidine 94
Cicatricial alopecia 166
Ciprofloxacin 230, 356
Clarithromycin 356
Clindamycin 68, 80, 102, 110, 118, 164, 168, 340
  topical 236
Clofazimine 270
Clotrimazole 10, 18, 46, 128, 180
Cloxacillin 88
Colchicine 94
Collodion flexile 176
Comedones 28, 293
Condyloma acuminata 218, 402
Contact dermatitis 170
  acute 8
  airborne 8, 16, 36, 96, 194, 202, 296, 388, 390
  irritant 178, 350
  pigmented 172
Corporis 18
Corticosteroids 54, 94, 202, 212, 204, 250, 266, 306, 322
  dose of 32
  intralesional 38, 60
  mid-potent 64
  potent 368

  topical 48
  superpotent 210, 274
  systemic 56, 308
  topical 386
Cotrimoxazole 248
Crisaborole 278, 346
Cruris 18
Cryosurgery 238
Cryotherapy 4, 90, 260, 272, 284, 290, 362, 402
Cutaneous drug reaction 342
Cyclophosphamide 108
Cyclosporine 160

D

Dapsone 94, 232, 248, 270
Dehydroepiandrosterone sulfate 153
Dental metal fitting 98
Dermatitis
  artefacta 66
  exfoliative 160
Dermatomyositis 34, 312
Dermatophytosis, recurrent 348
Dermatosis papulosa nigra 78
Dermographism 280
Dexamethasone 108
Diabetes, control of 58, 84, 272
Diabetic neurotrophic ulcer 366
Diphenylcyclopropenone 174
Discoid lupus erythematosus 166, 328, 368
Dithranol 210
Doxycycline 68, 82, 110, 190, 192, 222, 224, 236, 304, 340, 394
Dry lesions, chronic 177
Dyscrasias, hematological 308
Dyslipidemia
  management of 146
  screening for 146

E

Eczema 241, 338
  asteatotic 268
  chronic 338
  occupational hyperkeratotic 318
Eczematous lesions 169, 201, 204
Elbows 205
Electrocautery 260, 272, 284, 290, 362

Electrolyte balance 160
Electron beam 124
Electrosurgery 238
Emollients 44, 132, 216, 242, 268
    application 160
    liberal use of 178
Erythema
    heliotrope 33
    migrans 192
Erythematous follicular-based papules 375
Erythrasma 168
Erythroderma 160
    management of 160
Erythromycin 88, 168, 192, 230
Eumycetoma 248
External auditory meatus 106
Eye monitoring 246
Eyelids 189

F

Factitious cheilitis 320
Famciclovir 120
Fever, low-grade 239
Finasteride 76
Fixed drug eruption 14, 386
Flat-topped violaceous papules 311
Flexible collodion 72
Fluconazole 10, 18, 46, 128, 134, 152, 354
Fluid balance 160
Folliculitis 82
    decalvans 224
Footwear 202
    allergen of 202
Fordyce's granules 352
Fragile pustules 375
Fragrance 20, 132
Freckles 252
Free sebaceous glands 352
Furunculosis, recurrent 106
Fusidic acid 88, 224

G

Geographic tongue 180
Glans
    lichen planus of 324
    psoriasis on 158
Gliptin 226
Glomerulonephritis 88

Glucose-6-phosphate dehydrogenase screening 188
Glycolic acid 184
Gottron's papules 33
Granuloma pyogenicum 260
Groin 106

H

Hailey–Hailey disease 48
Hair dye 296
Hair loss
    female pattern 74, 198
    male pattern 76, 102
Halo nevus 196
Hamilton–Norwood type 76, 102
Hands
    knuckles of 33
    soap wash of 177
Hanseniasis 232
Herpes
    genitalis, recurrent 120
    labialis 314
    zoster 2
oticus 228
Hidradenitis suppurativa 138
Hirsutism 30, 214
Hopf acrokeratosis verruciformis 282
Hydroxychloroquine 166, 246, 368
Hygiene, maintenance of 18, 348
Hyperkeratosis, subungual 151
Hyperkeratotic lesions 175, 205, 301
Hypersensitivity
    insect 6
    syndrome 266
    vasculitis 316
Hypopigmentation over trunk 253
Hypothyroid 268

I

Iatrosacea 222
Ichthyosis vulgaris 52
Imiquimod 218, 402
Immunosuppressive 308
Impetigo
    cause of 88
    vulgaris 88
Infection
    bacterial 316
    control of 260

Inflammatory bowel diseases 308
Intertriginous eruption, recurrent 205
Isotretinoin 38, 80
Itching 3, 244
Itchy papules 249
Itchy papulovesicular lesions 305
Itraconazole 18, 46, 128, 134, 152, 248, 332, 354
Ivermectin 298

K

Keloid 4
Keratoacanthoma 364
Keratolytic 28
  mild 52
Keratosis pilaris 370
Ketoconazole 134, 220, 248
Knees 205
Kojic acid 184

L

Lactic acid 52, 72, 176
Lanolin 20, 132
Leg
  elevation 338
  ulcer, chronic 398
Lepromatous leprosy 270
Leprosy 12, 40
Lesions, perifollicular 133
Lichen
  amyloid 104
  nitidus 64
  planopilaris 56
  planus 10, 98, 324, 384
hypertrophicus 208
pigmentosus 112
  sclerosus et atrophicus 150, 372
  simplex chronicus 50
Light electrofulguration 78, 90, 148
Lignocaine 180, 390
Limbs, extensor surface of 215
Linear epidermal nevus 284
Linear morphea 276
Linezolid 106, 376
Lip
  balm 384, 386
  lichen planus of 384
Liver enzymes level 80
Loratadine 250

Luliconazole 18, 46, 128, 348, 354
Lymecycline 102, 110, 164, 340

M

Macrolides 68
Macules, pigmented 111
Maculopapular eruption, sudden-onset 211
Malar flush 245
Malignancy 254, 308
Malignant melanoma, development of 358
Mantoux test 99
Medication, Gliptin group of 304
Melanocytic nevus, congenital 358
Melasma 184
Meralgia paresthetica 122
Methotrexate 44, 210, 216
Metronidazole 68
  topical 68
Miconazole 168, 294
Miliaria rubra 360
Minocycline 164, 222, 224, 292, 308, 374
Minoxidil 76, 102, 154, 198
Moisturizer 322
Molluscum contagiosum 148, 238
Mometasone lotion 296
Morphea 60
Mucosa lesions 324
Multiple discharging
  sinuses 247
  ulcers 239
Mupirocin 88, 106, 118, 224, 376
Mycetoma 248
Mycobacteria, atypical 292
Mycobacterium tuberculosis 100
Mycophenolate mofetil 226, 304
Mycosis fungoides 124

N

Nail
  dystrophy 151
  pitting 209
Neurofibromatosis 130
Neurotic excoriation 344
Nevus
  depigmentosus 140
  spilus 26
Nikolsky's sign 107, 303

Nodular swelling 99
Nutrition care 160

O

Onychomycosis 152
Oxiconazole 128, 348, 354
Ozenoxacin 118, 224, 376

P

Pain 3, 299
  lignocaine for 180
  sudden-onset 227
Painful pustular lesions 117
Palmoplantar hyperhidrosis 114
Pancreatic carcinoma 262
Papillae, loss of 179
Papular urticaria 136
Papulosquamous skin eruption 189
Papulovesicles 5
Papulovesicular lesions 135
Paraben 20, 132
Para-phenylenediamine 61, 296
Parapsoriasis, small plaque 256
Parasitosis, delusion of 244
Paronychia, acute 288
Parthenium 96
Pasini atrophoderma 394
Patch testing 172, 296
Pemphigus
  erythematosus 32
  vulgaris 108, 400
Perifollicular inflammation 117
Perioral dermatitis 236
Periungual verruca 290
Permethrin 298
Phimosis, acquired 149
Photoallergic contact dermatitis 96, 194
Photosensitivity 245
Pierini atrophoderma 394
Pigmented purpuric dermatoses 200
Pimecrolimus 10, 68, 132, 158, 222, 278, 346, 378
Pityriasis
  alba 378
  lichenoides
    chronica 162
    et varioliformis acuta 326
  rubra pilaris 382
  versicolor 134, 220

Pityrosporum folliculitis 294
Plantar
  corn 176
  psoriasis 210
  verruca 72
Plaque psoriasis, chronic 206
Plasma cell 116
Podophyllin 402
Polycystic ovarian disease 101
Polymerase chain reaction 100
Polymorphous light eruption 186, 380
Pompholyx 204
Potassium dichromate 194
Povidone iodine shampoo 224
Prednisolone 40
Pregnancy, polymorphic eruption of 250
Prominent follicular keratosis 165
Propylene glycol application 52
Prurigo
  nodularis 274
  simplex 306
Pruritic erythematous eruption 7
Pruritic plaques, chronic 207
Pruritic vesicles, recurrent 203
Pruritus 131
Psoralen plus ultraviolet A therapy 124
Psoriasis 44, 158, 302
  flexural 206
  pustular 234
  vulgaris 216
Pyoderma gangrenosum 308

R

Ramsay Hunt syndrome 228
Retapamulin 88, 106
Rifampicin 40, 106, 232, 248, 270
Rosacea 68

S

Salicylic acid 52, 72, 104, 176, 210, 318
Scabies 258, 298
Scalp 189
  diffuse alopecia of 197
Scar 101
  management 80
Scleroderma
  localized 276
  systemic 86

Screening serum lipid profile 182
Scrofuloderma 240
Scrotal dermatitis 132
Scrotal skin 131
Scrotum 131
Sebaceous cyst 336
Senile acne 28
Serpiginous border 179
Sertaconazole 354
Sexually transmitted diseases 120, 218
Skin biopsy 108
Soft swelling 259
Squamous cell carcinoma 310
Staphylococcus aureus 360
Stasis dermatitis 20
Steroid 190
  acne 82
  low-potent topical 242
  modified tinea 332
  plus salicylic acid 302
  potent 178, 221
  systemic 92
  topical 162, 222
Streptomycin 248
Stress control 114, 132
Striae 70
Subcorneal pustular dermatoses 188
Sucralfate 94
Surgical circumcision 116
Swimming pool granuloma 292
Sycosis barbae 118
Syphilis, secondary 396
Systemic lupus erythematosus 34, 246

T

Tacrolimus 68, 96, 116, 132, 158, 196, 206, 278, 324, 346, 368, 378
Tap water iontophoresis 114
Tar 210
T-cell lymphoma, cutaneous 124
Terbinafine 18, 46, 128, 152
Tetracycline 94, 164, 190, 222, 224, 374
Throat infection 211
Thrombocytopenic purpura 156
Thrombophlebitis, recurrent 262
Tinea
  faciei 18, 128
  incognito 332
  pedis 46
  unguium 152
Tissue biopsy 100

Tretinoin 24, 28, 58, 70, 78, 84, 102, 164, 184
Triamcinolone, intralesional 4, 174, 208
Trichloroacetic acid 24, 72, 182
Trophic ulcer 12
True fungi 248
Truncal acne 340
Tuberculosis 240, 262

U

Ulcer 398
  care 308, 316
  proper dressing of 398
  regular dressing of 398
Ultraviolet B narrow band 62, 144
Umbilicus 106
Urethral dilatation 150
Urticaria, acute 92

V

Valacyclovir 22, 120, 314
Varicella 22
Verruca
  plana 24
  vulgaris 362
Vesicular dermatitis 204
Vesicular lesions, recurrent painful 119
Vitamin D analog 276
Vitiligo 144
  chemical 62, 330
  segmental 334

W

Wart 290
Weight, loss of 239
Whitish plaque, pattern of 97

X

Xanthelasma palpebrarum 182
Xanthoma, eruptive 146

Y

Yellowish-brown crust 87

Z

Zoon's balanitis 116

EU GSPR Authorised Reprsentative
Logos Europe, 9 rue Nicolas Poussin
1700, La Rochelle, France
Phone: +33 (0) 6 67 93 73 78
E-mail: contact@logoseurope.eu

www.ingramcontent.com/pod-product-compliance
Ingram Content Group UK Ltd.
Pitfield, Milton Keynes, MK11 3LW, UK
UKHW051137270226
468476UK00003B/19